Striving

for

Imprefection

per

Scott "Q" Marcus

THINspirational Columnist and Recovering Perfectionist

an additional
^52 Inspirational
Playful Columns
on Living Well,
Changing Habits,
and Other Acts of Faith

Striving for Imperfection
Volume 3

ISBN: 978-1466396562

Printed in the United States of America

For additional copies of this book, or to hire Scott "Q" Marcus for speaking,
training, consulting or workshops, call 707.442.6243
or scottq@scottqmarcus.com.

To get past what holds you or your business back,

go to www.ThisTimeIMeanIt.com

or

or www.ScottQMarcus.com

02.12.12

*Thanks to Mike Domitrz for the
inspiration, drive, and knowledge*

TABLE OF CONTENTS

Striving

for

Imprefection

per

Scott "Q" Marcus

THINspirational Columnist and Recovering Perfectionist

an additional
^52 Inspirational
Playful Columns
on Living Well,
Changing Habits,
and Other Acts of Faith

Thoughtful beginnings

If you were awake at 12:01AM January 2nd, you heard it. That giant CLUNK was the sound of the national psyche slamming over from "How much can I eat?" to "How quickly can I lose weight?" It happens every year at this time. Equally without fail is the inundation of advertisements, TV programs — and yes, columnists — who provide astute coaching on how to lose "those extra pounds" and get in shape. Warmed-over, threadbare, time-and-again guidance is ladled out in generous proportion each January, as reliably as winter rains. Chefs explain lower-fat meal preparation. Size zero models adorned in $500 leotards and $2000 running shoes champion their personal workout plans. Equally ubiquitous, snake oil infomercials attempt to pry consumer from wallet with assurances of medication and machines that "melt weight off without effort."

Been there, heard that. Over and over and over and over again…

I still weighed 250 pounds.

We know how to lose weight (eat less, be more active); it need not be belabored ad nausea. What blocks our progress is we just plain don't want to do it!

Yes, we desire good health. Yes, we like it when we look attractive. No, we are not fond of the stuffed-to-the-gills-can't-budge gastric distress following a binge of belly-busting burgers dripping with cheese and wrapped in pigful of bacon. The hitch in the get-along is that dieting takes forever; requires excessive, unending, Herculean, effort; and feels like it never succeeds. Why embark upon a laborious, frustrating voyage with defeat at its termination?

As said in college, "Flunk now, avoid the June rush."

When I started these weekly missives a few years back, I promised myself, the editors — and most important: YOU — that I would not dwell on "carbs, calories, and calisthenics;" that's everywhere already and we're not listening. Yes, nutrition and activity are essential to success, but what is lacking in the public dialogue is a conversation about the feelings, beliefs, and thoughts required for change.

We are not "food zombies," in control one moment, consuming uncountable calories the next, without some intervening thought process. In that illogical flash, I consider alternatives, rise from the couch, head to the kitchen, figure out what foods will comfort me — and only THEN do I drain the cabinets. I KNOW it's not healthy but this is not about smart, this is about feelings.

For the next few weeks, I'm doing a series: What goes into the heart and brain before whatever goes down the mouth and stomach. I.e. why do we do what we do when we know we won't like ourselves later? Whether you're trying to lose weight, stop smoking, or just change your attitude, I hope you enjoy.

Besides, at least for the time it takes to read 500 words, you won't be eating. And that's as good a start as any.

WHADYA WANT?

Note: This is the first in a five-part series on the mental and emotional adjustments required for long-term change

"People don't buy what they need, they buy what they want," so goes the age-old idiom used by sales trainers.

Some explanation is in order:

- "Buy" is not merely an exchange of currency for a product; "buy" can also be "make a decision" as in "buy into an idea." From such "mental purchases," actions result.

- We are not irrational; although "buying" begins emotionally, we back it with logic before finalizing the deal.

In other words, I might really, really, really want a bright red sporty convertible (can you say "mid life crisis?") but I then analyze my finances, examine my needs, and decide not to buy. However, if I don't "want" it first, I will not even weigh the options, so no purchase is possible.

Again: We buy what we want more than what we need; we back it with logic.

More germane to resolutions and habit change, I NEEDED to lose weight for years, yet it wasn't until my 39th birthday when I found myself eating leftover frosting from the pink cake box I had placed in the garbage, that I decided to actually do something.

Moreover, it was not that I even wanted to lose weight; in that moment all I wanted was to stop despising myself. I wanted control. I wanted to feel better. At that instant, I would do virtually anything to make the pain stop. Born from that strong emotional state, I only then analyzed my options and alternatives — and moved forward.

Change is generated by fear, force, or pain — not happiness. If life were idyllic with butterflies, flowers, and sunshine greeting each morning, why would any-one want to change? However, from the fire of ache, desires arise; the paradox being that once that hurt starts to recede (or the reality of the effort sets in) I no longer WANT to do the work as it appears laborious, tedious, and non-productive. I revert to familiar easier habits, figuring "there's always tomorrow." Therein lies the seed of every broken resolution.

To break that cycle, one must focus on what is GAINED from the effort, not what is sacrificed. Weight loss is NOT about abandoning favorite foods; it's about feeling in control. It is NOT about grunting and panting through an exercise program, it's about enjoying freedom of movement. Each is true, one we WANT — and move toward it; the other we don't — we steer away.

To make change permanent, it is imperative that we focus on its benefits. It's still a long road but a more productive, positive, and exciting path.

BELIEVE IT

Second in a series on the mental and emotional adjustments required for long-term change

The famous early-twentieth century escape artist, Harry Houdini, traveled the countryside, locking himself in jails, only to escape, as a method of furthering his reputation (and increasing his audiences). As the story goes, there was only one chamber from which he could not free himself.

Houdini entered the fateful cell and began his usual routine once the iron bars clanged shut. From his belt, he removed a concealed piece of metal utilized to pick locks, and set about as he had done countless times before. Whereby every previous security device had soon swung open, he could not achieve the desired results on this occasion.

Finally, after laboring for hours, bathed in sweat and exhausted, Houdini collapsed in frustration against the cell door, defeated. As he fell against it, it swung wide — it was unlocked the entire time.

Because Houdini believed he was trapped, he was. So too are we ensnared by our beliefs.

If I do not believe I can lose "those extra pounds," all the forces of Heaven and Earth cannot force success upon me. It matters not the number of "experts" and self-help gurus who ply me with easy-to-follow step-by-step instructions, exercise plans, or medical research.

As example, if after losing 12 pounds, I have a temporary setback of two pounds, I will see that as validation of what I already "knew": that I cannot lose weight.

"It was only a matter of time," I'll say to myself. "I knew it couldn't last."

Beliefs influence feelings; therefore defeated and despondent, I think, "Why am I wasting my time?" From thoughts come actions; in this case that would be getting off the scale, tossing my diet materials in the trash, and deciding to give up for now. I revert to old habits. My losses evaporate, my bulks returns.

The final consequence is my beliefs are again validated and the cycle resumes.

The reality about weight loss is that it is not a linear downward progression, even for the ultra dedicated and diligent. Rather, it is a learned skill, trial and error. Successful weight loss is actually losing more weight than one gains; down four pounds, up one, down three, up two. (Picture a stock market chart from a downward Bear market and you get an accurate concept.)

If my belief is that periodic gains are part of the process, I will still feel frustrated and saddened by the setback, but shall continue the course, possibly making some corrections. Two pounds are two pounds; resulting actions differ only because underlying beliefs do.

What we say to ourselves become our beliefs; if they work, they are of value to us. If not, it is vital we change them.

Believe me.

Shrinking it down

Third in a series on the mental and emotional adjustments required for long-term change

I believe in the basic goodness of people.

Because of that, my feelings towards most are benevolent; I cut people some slack, assist the downtrodden when possible, and experience a general contentedness with life. The result is, on the whole, people treat me well and I feel fortunate. (Although I periodically forget, so you might need to remind me.)

Because I believe, I act. Actions cause results, which feed into — or work against — my beliefs. In that process is another of the great circles of life.

Beliefs are the bedrock of who we are — and who we become. To a large extent, they determine whether we live well, the quality of our relationships, and even our connection with God and the Universe. Powerful forces, they are not to be reckoned with lightly.

Beliefs: closely held values accepted as facts and validated by observation, are the essential component in lifestyle change. It is hard to look in the mirror while weighing 250 pounds and have faith that "this time" I will be successful, when in fact, all previous attempts merely ended as failure, leaving me weighing more now than I ever have previously. If I do not believe, it matters not how many experts tell me to eat less and be more active. In my mind, I know I will not succeed and will therefore see failure, not setbacks; defeat, not delay. I will quit.

I was not born believing that I would always be fat; that took time to develop. As a child, my parents, concerned about my size, stressed its dangers. Doctors put me on thousand-calorie diets with purple-ink mimeographs and lists of low calorie foods. My clothes came from the "husky" section. Boys teased me; girls avoided me. Each time I was impeded in my diet, internal voices screeched, "See, you can't change; it's impossible!" I stopped, further validating my beliefs.

Beliefs can and do change. What's counter intuitive is that process happens not by thinking big, but small. One's life is not constructed in years, rather via minutes and seconds. Small, almost imperceptible ticks of the clock come together to make me who I am, leaving behind who I was. It is almost imperceptibly slow, but is happening — even now.

When I no longer looked at 70 pounds — or even ten — as the validation of success, changes began. Instead of the "whole thing," I targeted five pounds, or three, sometimes even one. At times, success was getting through the next five minutes.

Each slight triumph — if focused upon — became an in-your-face defiance of the old guard, knocking down its structure, brick-by-brick, girder by ledger.

To adjust beliefs, concentrate on minor victories. They will get larger when given their due.

STAMINA OVER SPEED

Last in a special series on the mental and emotional adjustments required for long-term change

Anyone could tell she was annoyed with the result. Although she lost weight from the previous week, her irritation was palpable.

"One quarter of a pound? Four lousy ounces!" She continued to stare at the scale. "I exercised. I wrote everything down; I even stayed away from the hors d'oeuvres at the office party. This is too slow. I won't hit my right weight until I'm 60!"

Standing down from the platform, I heard her grumble as she snatched her purse, "Who needs this frustration?" With those final words, she stormed from the meeting. The next time she came to a meeting, she weighed 43 pounds more than when she had left — and was three years closer to the "dreaded" age of sixty.

At times it is difficult to remember that "slower is faster than never."

Few events are more exasperating than diligently following a plan, faithfully monitoring your efforts, expecting breathtaking rewards, and ending up feeling punished for the effort. Hope vanishes, motivation evaporates, and the seductive siren song of harmful habits slyly lures us off track. After all, rarely does one give up when all is doing well.

Success requires enduring many such indignities; it involves making a lifestyle — not temporary — change. Logically, we know that "lifestyle change" must last… well, er, um … a lifetime (hence the term).

Emotionally however, we want to experience all the payback without making the required investment. As a further analogy, we crave the benefits of wisdom without enduring the exposure to life.

It does not work that way. The process will not be rushed; it must be fully experienced.

Success is more likely when we understand the benefits begin immediately; we do not have to wait to enjoy them until we get "there." To the contrary, that magical land where temptation is non-existent and motivation is ever present is fantasy; there is no better prescription for failure than betting the farm on such unrealistic expectations.

Those who obtain their goals are still faced with the same temptations and frustrations as those of us still striving for our objectives. What differs is they persevere through rough periods by changing focus, not by ignoring the delay.

Setbacks cannot be avoided. Although it might not feel so in the moment, each one presents an opportunity to understand the process, ourselves, and make the adjustments necessary for long-term, SUSTAINED change.

At those crossroads, look back, not ahead. The future is always unknown, yet the road already traveled — no matter how short the journey — is lined with accomplishments: some small, others more significant.

Motivation returns when the focus changes.

THE PIXIE DUST DIET

Those sparkling, glittering, glowing flecks I have scattered on you cause no harm; do not be alarmed. It is pixie dust from whence great magic comes.

Immediately great wealth beyond all expectation will befall you! Vary not your customary routine; dollars will gravitate to you. Strangers will bestow upon you copious quantities of currency. A gold vein will be unearthed in your backyard. Congress will declare a new tax with all proceeds delivered to an account of your choosing.

That is merely the beginning.

Not only will these gleaming granules of glorious glitter augment your bottom line, they impart supernatural powers. While holding a few flecks, click together your heels three times, spin twice to the east, sing passionately your favorite show tune, and you will become as the breeze and elevate weightlessly into the sky, able to fly with the birds along the tops of redwoods.

These miniscule specks also possess extraordinary healing power. You will live countless years in perfect health. Nothing unpleasant will befall you; disease is non-existent, accidents a concern of the past.

Live boldly. Live large; for you have been infused with the powder of pixies.

I detect cynicism; how can you doubt? We are exposed to countless similar claims of buffoonery proclaiming equally implausible benefits, all wrapped in the blanket of the "latest secret of weight loss". Why do we believe those, yet scoff at equally implausible payback of pixie powder?

One supplement on line proclaims, "a total body makeover pill for women of all ages," and professes to suppress appetite, enlarge breast tissue, and super charge your sex drive. (Who would have known that bust size is related to weight loss?) I'm sure this miracle of modern medicine even cleans the house, helps students with calculus, and solves geopolitical struggles in the Middle East on weekends. Such claims are similarly believable.

Another product is cloaked in ancient mysteries, declaring to reveal "The Secret" from ancient scrolls containing "many little-known health and weight loss secrets, including a fountain of youth-like philosophy called 'lean-gevity.'" Should we mere mortals have a chance to peruse these scrolls, they probably read, "eat less, move more, and focus on long-term change." However, such details are omitted from the on-line marketing materials — must be an oversight. No worry however; for merely $79, one can share the enlightenment. I cannot get my credit card at the ready quickly enough.

I so often wish I could pop a pill, read a scroll, or swallow a concoction that would magically change the traits I do not like about myself. Alas, I do live in reality; no products will ever accomplish those goals. However, achieving results through self-control, determination, and healthy choices is a magical feeling.

IN THREE WEEKS

They say, "Eat less and exercise more; the weight will practically fall off." They also say, "getting started is the hardest part." Of course, garrulous as They are, They make sure to point out you shouldn't have waited so long before taking care of yourself. Whoever "They" are, They sure have a lot to say about how to run your life, don't They?

They also tell you that if you keep a new habit in place for only three weeks, it will be adapted into your life. I'm not sure I agree. I've been dieting since before they invited sugar-free cola and non-fat yogurt — considerably more than three weeks — and I still find healthy eating a challenge, especially when stressed with organizing my taxes, calling the plumber to fix a plugged toilet, and trying to find a few seconds for my family. In those moments, a double-bacon, cheesy, chili burger and gargantuan order of fries still shout pretty loud.

Yet, if you have ever tried to adjust habits, you have faced the dreaded (insert ominous music here…) "Three Week Barrier."

In Week One, all is new and exciting. You are inspired (or at least willing) to do what it takes; after all, you've stopped putting it off, might as well get on with the task at hand. Once the decision has finally been made, activity begins; changes occur; motivation results.

By Week Two — if you look for it — you see a few fledgling results. Even though the path ahead appears long, these early outcomes keep you plodding onward.

At Week Three, most people start facing as many setbacks as successes. As Life is wont to do, it throws some curves, and dealing with these stresses generates the urge for comfort, in effect the desire to revert to old habits. Confronted with instantaneous chocolate gratification or what appears a tortuous, arduous, uphill life-long slog, most opt to "try again later, when things finally settle down." (Not wishing to be morbid, but I must point out the only time things "finally settle down," your weight won't matter to anyone but the six friends carrying you to your final resting place.)

If it is accurate that every person faces frustrations, why do some persevere while others fall victim to the lure of the old ways?

I'm glad you asked. While some focus on external results, craving to "get there quickly" so we can "stop thinking about this all the time," others direct their attention to their feelings when confronted with these inevitable setbacks. They remind themselves of the successes so far, meager as they might seem. Although frustrated, they slow down long enough to learn from the feedback, and work on adjusting their attitude — even if only for an instant. Without ongoing fine-tuning, we are condemned to repeat old patterns.

PARADOXES

Why do we treat with disdain that which we love?

That sounds like sappy dialogue from a poorly penned science-fiction movie — a supposedly wise paradox accepted as profound philosophy; while in reality, a load of cheap gibberish gussied up in cut-rate fabric and touted as Sunday finery.

"One must live in darkness to truly see light."

That is silliness, nothing more. However there are paradoxes of serious concern. As example, there is no greater joy than the excitement, enthusiasm, and absolute elation derived from the self-control of beating back one's personal demons. When I turn down an extra helping of potato salad; ride my bike when I would rather drive; or opt for healthy food over junk; an infusion of vitality and confidence electrifies my soul unlike any other sensation. Should it be possible to bottle and distribute that sentiment, Heaven itself would pale in comparison to life on Earth.

So, why do I fight that euphoria which I adore so much? Am I resistant to joy? It is there, patiently waiting for the taking, always within reach; ready to embrace me. Yet I so often turn away.

I set up my day to run behind schedule, thereby forcing myself to avoid the reduced stress and enhanced feeling of fitness that I receive when I walk on my errands. I contort and twist my mental processes to rationalize an excuse giving me permission to finish a bag of tortilla chips, knowing that revulsion that will overcome me later.

It is a paradox of sad proportion. I have within me the ability to feel fantastic, emboldened, and fulfilled; or I can opt for the lowly pathway of immediate gratification and the grief that follows. That which I find irresistible, I avoid. That which I detest, I embrace.

In most of my life, I "do what it takes." I (usually) make choices necessary for closeness with my family, which might not always be the easiest option. To enhance my career, I force myself to face the scary places, make the cold calls, take the risks. Yet, in this one part of my life — one that means so very much — I take the short cuts.

In college, I learned a proverb; "When all is perfect, the Gods become jealous of you and therefore take something away." Have I set up my life to leave one component a kilter to keep those Gods at bay? Moreover, the irony is that when we do exercise the will and control within — even for mere moments — we are more in touch with all that is holy and glorious than at any other time; a thought worth remembering the next time Choice comes calling.

THE BREAK UP

Relationships come and go but I have been deeply involved with calories for a very long time. We were not smarties, rather a couple of chunky dum-dum nerds on a rocky road: snickering together, exchanging chocolate kisses. Sweet things were left for me each day and I was wooed by those charms. I went goo-goo over the relationship.

Our time was good — and plenty. Periodically, we escaped for extended cross-country excursions, enjoying each other on Fifth Avenue as we traversed that long, licorice highway, viewing the Milky Way, admiring Mars. I remember one particular trip where we spent the night on a farm, treated by a jolly rancher. I have to tell you, he was a lifesaver.

Calories came to my workplace, offering sage advice, spicing up my day. When frustrated and angered by writer's block, I ventured to the kitchen for consultations with chocolates and cookies. When I returned, gone was Mr. Chip from my shoulder, leaving me filled again, dissatisfaction in peeces. But I don't need to explain that, u-know how it is when you're on a roll.

By the glow of a flickering TV screen, after payday, I sat with potato crisps, tortilla chips, and candy. Not a peep would be uttered, I could tell simply by the look that I was wanted and needed, like a big hunk.

However, I am finding that our relationship — although very filling — is causing me heartache (and heartburn). I have been trying to fudge how I feel but I must consider moving on. I am afraid I might be turning into a sucker.

Oh sure, we had great times. I will long for midnight rendezvous in the kitchen, finding passion with leftover mashed potatoes and cold cuts to the soft light of an open refrigerator. Rainy Sundays coupled with croissants and scones made for great times; I won't be able to peruse the morning paper without crying, especially when I read the recipe page.

It is important to understand I have no beef with this relationship and I am not chicken to move forward. I just want to make sure what I do is well done. So it is with heavy heart and heavier waistline that I have come to this fork in the road, indeed an irony, since that utensil has usually been party to more positive moments. I have so many mixed feelings; having to fold-in many thoughts, beating and whipping myself up, egging myself onward, processing and blending all we have been. My concern is how this will pan out.

This decision should be easy as pie, yet it is no cakewalk. What I do know is that it is eating me alive and I better make up my mind, before I waist any more time.

THE VOICES

A fierce battle rages within me each time unexpected goodies are offered my way.

Let me set up a scenario. I stop by Jim's office to pick up a flyer. Cake, brownies, and pie are strewn about the table in the employee lounge. He says, "We had a party in Brenda's honor today. Help yourself."

We now join the internal conversation, already in progress…

Voice number one: "Wow! Look at all those goodies. Go for it!"

Voice number two (the skinny one): "It's merely food Scott! It's not like you've never had chocolate cake before. Get a grip!"

V1: "But it's free. That makes it better."

V2: "It still has calories. Just because you don't pay for it doesn't mean it won't make you fat."

V1: "Ah, come on. Don't be a stick in the mud. It's just going to go to waste if you don't eat it. Think of all the starving people who would jump at a chance for this much food."

V2: "Just because it could be wasted doesn't make me the garbage disposal. And, as for the starving people, I can donate to Food for People. But, if I eat this, they don't gain weight — I do."

V1: "OK, appealing to your sense of global values isn't going anywhere. Let's try this. How do you feel when you spend a whole lot of time looking for that perfect gift for your wife, and then she opens it, and you can tell by the look in her eyes that she's disappointed?"

V2: "Let down, a little sad I guess."

V1: "Right. And then you get distant from her. And she pulls back. And soon you're having an argument about something that's totally unrelated, like the toothpaste cap or the time you didn't clean the grill when she asked you to."

V1: "What's your point?"

V2: "Well, it's kind of like that, see? Jim and you are good friends as well as business associates, right?"

"Yes, so?"

"So, he's thinking of you by offering a chance to share in the celebration of his workmate. By providing these treats, he's really saying, 'We don't spend enough time together socially. I'm trying to make up for that by giving you these goodies. Please don't turn your back on me. I'm feeling very vulnerable right now.'"

"All that is involved in this? I thought he was just being friendly."

"Don't be naive, men aren't good at discussing emotions so it comes out other ways."

"Well I wouldn't want to hurt his feelings. I guess a little bit is OK."

As I reach for the plate, Jim says, "Oh yeah, I've been meaning to talk to you. You do so well watching your weight. I was hoping for a few tips."

My hand lurches to the right and I pour a cup of coffee instead, only to hear myself reply, "It's simple actually. Just follow your inner voice."

HISTORY

Purchased from the Thomas Page company for "$100 in gold coin" on "lot 7 of block 7", and constructed of redwood in 1907, the Church of the Oaks in Cotati, California, has been in the same location on the corner of Page and West Sierra since its construction. The one room, unimposing, white building has watched over this town from its grassy lot for 100 years.

Prior to the service where I would speak to the small congregation, I sat noiselessly in the modest, tranquil sanctuary, infused with the presence of a century of people who sat where I was now. Some lives began here; others heard their final tribute; now the life-energy of each was as much a part of this building as its stained glass windows or bell tower.

Within these hardy, dark, handcrafted, timber walls, I imagined Edna Meriwether given in holy matrimony to William Johnson, encircled by the local gathering of family and friends. The church bell chimed a joyous noise that echoed through the small burg; while outside, next to the magnificent oak, the sound of fiddles, dancing, and carefree conversation drifted through the trees.

Sarah Williamson listened to the minister as he eulogized the premature passing of her husband, Jonah, when his tractor rolled on him while he plowed the fields one foggy morning during the 1930s. He had tilled the same patch of earth since he was a boy. This spot where Emmanuel, their son, had been baptized, was Jonah's last stop before he was lowered into the Earth.

The flock sought solace in this place during times of urgency. Sermons of spiritual import were delivered from its pulpit as it listened intently with somber understanding. It rejoiced to banjo music on weekend dances; and was uplifted by hymns of praise at Sunday service.

The church stood witness to it all. Although constructed of redwood and bound together by nails and screws, these walls reflected the heart of a community. If one listened, one could hear the beating, rhythmic, pulsing, formed over decades.

Each of us is a sanctuary of our own past. We are not simply what we our present; but we carry within all that has come before, from unlimited voices and countless decisions. We each hold dear a rich history, some of it unfortunate, some truly glorious. Yet it is all came together to where we stand now. Every past choice, whether correct or in error, set us upon a path to today. Whether good or bad or in between, we cannot return.

Yet, we are not locked at this time. Each and every choice we make today will become our history tomorrow.

POINT OF VIEW

Due to a recent bout of unexpected sunshine, I was persuaded to abandon the comfort of our couch to work in our yard. Although my wife's and my relationship is quite balanced, she has deemed lawn upkeep as "Scott's job." I know not why, as I have not requested this high honor, and, to be quite frank, am not particularly skilled in this arena. Nonetheless, being her loving pawn, I march duly forth with lawn mower and weed eater to engage the high grass.

Our lot is not particularly large, unless one is faced with the prospect of mowing it… and the grass is long — and wet; three intertwined dynamics of last weekend. This permutation of factors means I cannot simply drag the mower over my property once; rather I must set the cutter to maximum height, labor to and fro, back and forth across the bumpy lawn (periodically grinding to a stop on uneven clumps of mud), shake the bulky, heavy, dismally designed bag with the ridiculously narrow opening numerous times, then repeat, repeat, repeat. After this preliminary trimming, I lower the cutter and engage in this funfest yet again.

While attempting to stuff the gooey, wet, stinky, clippings into the lawn bag, it rips and falls, spilling a mess along the sidewalk. I now grab the push broom (a tool close to useless for sweeping wet, sticky grass from asphalt) and proceed to sweep (such as it is) and scoop the grass back into the sack, only to have it yet again tumble (this time to the other side), spilling even more of its contents, changing my routine from sweep and scoop, to sweep, scoop, and swear.

Whether triggered by the pain in my back, the sun in my eyes, or the sweat soaking my brow, I do not know; yet a random thought skipped across my mind as I bent down to lift the green waste, "At least I'm not shoveling show in freezing temperatures. THAT would be a major drag."

And in that instant, lifting wet grass in overfull, black, heavy lawn bags seemed a lot better. How can I complain about maintaining my very own front yard, in a good neighborhood, on a mild day — and being healthy enough to do it — when so many cannot even afford a mortgage? And what about those who simply wish for a roof over their head? In that light, I'm blessedly fortunate.

With that thought as a launch-off point, I realized again that point of view is essential. Many go to bed with distended stomachs and hunger pains, and I so quickly lament that my double Grande extra hot latte has to have non-fat instead of whole milk, or that I must bypass ordering a chocolate muffin to accompany it.

Funny, huh? Look one way; life stinks; look another's it's mighty fine. (I will still admit however that it would a gardener would make it even a little better.)

COLORING
BOOKS AND COMMITMENTS

I was "row monitor" in second grade; sitting in the last seat, making sure all students in row #4 behaved. If not, their name was recorded in my official "monitor's notebook," which at day's end, was delivered to the teacher. Right now, during daily quiet time, everyone was behaving appropriately. No one messed with the law when I was on duty.

If all was calm, and we had no pending assignments, we were given permission to color. Each of us had a coloring book in our desk for just such occasion. Eagerly, I pulled my precious book from inside my desk and began flipping through the pages, looking for just the right picture. I always colored the "way cool" pictures first, usually images with robots or ray guns. Alas, they were all completed. Slightly disappointed, but undaunted, I dropped to the next level, the boring pictures - the ones with horses or girls in them.

"Make a mental note," I told myself, "get a new coloring book – no girl pictures." But since that was all that remained, I began flipping pages. Nothing. The entire coloring book was full.

Sadly, I slid my book into its home, folded my hands on my desk, looked up at the clock, sighed, and waited; I had absolutely nothing to do.

I believe that was the last time I remember that happening.

Back then; there was more time than I could ever fill. Its vast landscape stretched out unbroken in front of me forever, no urgency, a million tomorrows yet to come. To a child, there seems no end point, no termination; life is a road without finish. Anything is possible whenever one should choose.

My life today is poles apart from how it was when I was seven. Now, I pay considerable sums of money to take cruises, putting me in a place where I force myself to do "nothing." Like an addict going through withdrawal, the first few days without assignments and deadlines feel awkward and uncomfortable. Finally, when I can settle down and relax, I become tense over my pending return to the garble of assignments and responsibilities that cascade through my waking hours, keeping me amped from before dawn to after dark.

In a world crushed by deadlines and everyday jobs, we too often delay Responsibility One: taking care of ourselves so we can enjoy this ride as long as possible.

"One of these days," I will get my act together. "Someday soon," I will eat correctly, "When the time is right," I will spend more time with my family.

We — like the wide-eyed children we no longer are — feel there's constantly tomorrow, still another sunrise to come. That might be. However, there is no guarantee.

Why not begin today?

Now, where did I put that coloring book?

IN AN INSTANT

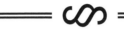

It is not over years, but in an instant that everything changes.

Elizabeth Edwards, wife of presidential candidate, John Edwards, and a powerful figure of her own accord, has had a reoccurrence of breast cancer, metastasizing in her bones. One minute, she's "cancer-free," the next moment, she is facing a decision that could be of historic proportions for our country.

So much happens in one tick of a clock.

Tony Snow, White House press spokesman, enters the hospital for a "routine" procedure to remove a growth from his abdomen. It is a safe bet to assume that day turned out to be anything but "routine" for the Snow family.

Two political figures, with widely disparate views, are at once united in a battle against a common enemy; a poignant reminder that more binds us than drives us apart. It matters not what one owns, or the power one wields, mortality is unimpressed by stature.

It goes without saying that not only the rich and powerful, or those with access to our national spotlight must face their moments. Each of us, is — or will be — confronted with "instants" that upend everything we know. (I pray for the courage of Ms. Edwards when mine comes.)

These national events, coupled with cheerless news from some friends, have brought to the surface emotions I prefer to avoid, yet apparently, cannot. I hold little fear of heart attack or stroke. I do (most of) what I can to avoid their cold grasp: I eat well; engage in moderate, regular, exercise; and have years (and years) of therapy to cope with the psychological and emotional ravages that might trigger such events.

Cancer, however, is a far different story. The very word slams a stake of terror through my heart.

My mother was a victim of that wretched, abominable, scourge; dragging her from diagnosis to death in 18 blindingly short days — an instant. It was an horrific, dreadful period where we helplessly watched her decline from what we thought was healthy, vibrant, and active; to her demise. Seven years hence, it remains a gaping tear in the fabric of my life.

Yet, although I still bitterly miss her, and feel deeply for others facing such challenges, I believe with utter certainty that it is a travesty to park myself idly and fearfully by the side of life's road, waiting for whatever fate shall bring. Death may be natural, but avoiding Life is sinful.

Until that moment when I have no options, I still retain some control. In any fragment of time — including this very second — I must therefore remind myself to inhale deeply the beauty of all that surrounds me; smile more often at the pleasures I possess; and honor those who no longer have those options by infusing myself, totally, and completely with the Spirit of Health and Wellbeing that I still possess in THIS instant.

Speeding through life

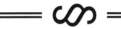

The very first time I sat in the therapist's office, my initial question was not in search of personal insights, philosophical uplift, nor deep understanding. Rather it was a rudimentary and mundane query, "How long will this take?"

Glancing at his watch, he glibly replied, "About 50 minutes."

"No," I countered, "I mean how long before I am fixed?"

"First of all," he said, "You're not broken; you do not need to be fixed. The thing about mental health is that you understand you will never completely 'get your act together;' you develop tools that help you handle better the problems you face and enjoy your life more in the process. However, once you deal with the surface issues, others will come to view; so in a manner of speaking, one never gets there. Shall we begin?"

Forty-nine minutes to go; this was going to be a very long hour.

Since then, I have indeed learned quite a lot:

One: I make positive choices more often than I don't.

Two: Despite knowing the correct thing to do — I do not always opt to do so. (However, one those occasions when I choose to "walk off a cliff," there is some small measure of satisfaction in at least knowing I am making a choice, and not merely a victim of random circumstance.)

Three: I still want to rush the process so I can be "there" already. At times, I tire of self-analysis and deep thought. I simply expect the Universe to operate the way I think it should. What's wrong with that?

As illustration, I wish I could lose those "extra pounds" without having to change any habits. That way, I could stop thinking about calories, carbs, and calisthenics every blasted waking minute. Then — I promise — I will lead a 100% healthy lifestyle and maintain this new body. It's not like I don't know how; so what use is there in undergoing this torturous, monotonous process of yet again? I swear I have learned my lesson. Just get me to the destination and I'll prove it.

Insanity is described as "doing the same thing over and over and expecting a different result." If I am indeed seeking physical and mental health; and every time I follow the "hurry-up-and-get-there path," I regain my weight; maybe a thought adjustment is required.

Those things of which I am most proud (physically, emotionally, and spiritually) all came from effort. I saved money, educated my mind, and developed my beliefs. Setbacks, although unpleasant, were the genesis for understanding and growth.

If life is a journey and not a destination, why race for the end? I lament how quickly my days pass, yet disregard the present, urgently longing for tomorrow, sacrificing the only actual time I have: Now.

Maybe if I can enjoy today, tomorrow will be even better.

Now Boarding

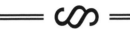

It is more convenient to take a trip to a convention center to speak to 300 people than it is to cram them all in my living room. Therefore I spend a goodly share of time in airports. Although there are many kind and respectable people employed within, I often find myself irritated with the process of getting from where I am to where I wish to be, specifically the lines, security, and all-too-common delays.

This frustration — coupled with the need to arrive for my flight before even the sun is awake — causes me to not sleep well the night prior to my travels. Because I am paranoid about being late, I plan to rise at 4AM, which will provide enough time to clear security, check in, and stagger over to the local barrista so he can jump-start my heart with excessive doses of caffeine. To make sure I actually do rise at such an inhumane hour, I set an alarm clock, cell phone, and PDA. (Should all three blare at the same instant, I would probably suffer a heart attack from the unexpected cacophony and miss my flight anyway.)

Reality is alarms are unnecessary because I toss and turn through the night, afraid to oversleep. The internal insomniac conversation is akin to this:

2:00 AM: "I'm going to be so exhausted tomorrow. C'mon Scott, relax! Fall asleep NOW!"

2:30 AM: "OK, if I pass out this second, I can still get 90 minutes; I can get by on that."

3:00 AM: "I'll sleep on the plane and take a ten minute nap between presentations. Cats get by on short naps, why can't I?"

3:15 AM: "Sleep is over-rated. Maybe I should just get up. I'll drink lots of coffee."

3:30 AM: "Oh, forget it! What's the use? I might as well get moving."

With that thought, I drop my feet over edge of the bed and drag my exhausted body into the shower, hoping to revitalize myself enough to get to the airport before collapsing in the arms of Hypnos, the God of Sleep.

As I recently lie restlessly in the darkness, I thought, "At which point do I finally decide to face the inevitable, get up, and get moving?" I know how this is going to turn out; I might as well accept it. What causes me to finally cross that line? When do I shift from inactivity to realization to action? I squander so much time forcing myself into stagnation, knowing all the while the outcome is predestined. Denial and delay are not successful strategies.

This routine, I decided, is a metaphor for much of life. As frustration mounts and the inevitability of what needs to be done pushes ever closer, we find unlimited rationales to avoid doing what we'll eventually do any-way. "There's always later." "Problem, what problem?" "Ignore it and it will go away."

The alarm is blaring; the destination awaits; all seats are boarding. Check your baggage, it's time to go.

Miracle Diet

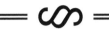

"I lost 18 pounds my first 24 hours while still enjoying chocolate, French fries, and beer! The best thing is it's been a whole day and I haven't gained back a pound!"

Hard to believe, isn't it? Like millions of women, Zelda Smith, always fought the battle of the bulge.

"Since I was young, I was chubby. Other kids made fun of me, teasing me and embarrassing me on the playground. As an adult, it only got worse."

"It didn't matter what I did, weight just kept piling on. I tried everything, switching to low-fat foods, watching what I ate; I even stopped using chocolate syrup as salad dressing. At meals, I tried limiting myself to only what could fit on one plate, never going back for seconds. My sister — who's never been supportive — scoffed. She said, 'Zelda, if you're going to do the one-plate thing, I don't think you should use a platter. It defeats the purpose.' Do you see what I've had to put up with?"

"But I didn't let her deter me; I was determined! So I adjusted my lifestyle. I went to the gym; I even got out of my car and went inside once. At home I exercised regularly — ten minutes once a month, just like clockwork. I found other ways to increase my activity. I started walking to the mailbox instead of driving; my husband really appreciated that because he found it hard to get in the front door when I left the car parked on the porch. Sometimes, when I was really inspired, I even put down the remote control and walked all the way over to the TV to shut it off. It's not easy to change your life, but when something's worth it, you sacrifice."

"Still, I was frustrated by the lack of results. So I went to one of those weight loss support groups. I thought I was going to die the first time I walked in the meeting, listening to that skinny young thing talk about how she lost weight by using some silly fad diet involving eating right and exercising. I thought, 'No way this will work!' But, I took the materials home and bought a food scale and put them right over there — in that drawer — where they've been for six months. You would think after that long, I would have lost something, wouldn't you? See, nothing works."

"Then, I discovered the new Placebo Sham Diet with miracle additive Cleanyouout! Wow! I take one pill every hour with a cup of castor oil, six raw eggs, and their patented ingredient, "laxital," and — Voila! — the weight just drops off you. Of course, it helps to be near the rest room when it takes effect, but 18 hours a day in the bathroom is a small price to pay for a size five body. Someday soon, I'm hoping to get out of here and show it to everyone!"

The only diet that works?

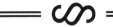

I'm really getting too old for this as my knees are getting a little worn; however, I cannot shirk my public responsibility; I must yet scale again my towering soapbox and speak truth to power.

Extra! Extra! Researchers at UCLA say dieting doesn't work!

Yep, according to some of the most advanced minds medical science can cobble together in a laboratory, a recent study discovered that people lose weight initially, but many relapse and regain their weight. In other words, losing weight is easy; keeping it off — not so much.

In the "tell-me-something-I-don't-already-know" department, an obesity researcher at USC added, "It's difficult to modify your diet and turn away from the pleasures of eating." Uh, hello? We didn't know this? Thanks pal for shedding light on that big deep, dark, hidden, mystery. Science marches on.

As I read further, what did my eyes spy but this line: "Specialists generally agree that surgery is the only proven method to keep weight off."

My, oh my, oh my! Where do I even begin? Surgery: the ONLY proven method? Have we lost complete touch with what we're discussing?

This exemplifies the misguided quick fix thinking that surrounds weight loss. Of course, it's a given that extreme plans will fail. If all one does is draw a line in time and say, "Henceforth, I shall never again eat those foods," or conversely, "Those are the only foods I will eat," (the traditional patterns of many diets) the result is a fiasco as "the dieter" is not dealing with the actual cause of her problem: it is NOT what she eats, rather how she thinks.

Our actions — overeating — are not random zombie-like impulses. They are always preceded by thought; sometimes that spark is so blindingly quick (read "habit"), it goes unnoticed, yet it is without exception the pre-cursor. Therefore, if we don't change how we think — what we say to ourselves — we are forever condemned to repeat the offending actions causing weight gain. So, the report is accurate in that, "Most people will put their weight back on." However, it is not due to lack of surgery or powerlessness; rather the frustrating cycle is because we do not focus on doing the inner work necessary for long-term success.

There are some times when surgery is indeed needed, but have we become so addicted to scalpels and pills that we simply toss in the trash heap the phenomenal abilities of the human spirit and drive?

We are miraculous creatures, capable of breath-taking works of art, mu-sic that heals the soul, and words that move nations. We have created towering structures that stroke the heavens, machines that breathe life into the dying, and vehicles that can be hurled billions of miles across the vast expanse of space, landing within a bull's-eye the size of my back yard. Surely we are capable of saying, "No thank you" to an extra serving of key lime pie, closing our mouth, and enjoying the success of accomplishment.

It doesn't take surgery for that.

I'M PROUD OF YOU

His energy reminded me of a tightly coiled spring, overloaded with caffeine, bouncing on a trampoline. Of course, most three-year-old children do not walk in an even, orderly, refined gait, and he was no exception; bouncing and bounding in a generally forward direction, yet so easily distracted by the zip and zing of the airport. Although secured to mom by a strap attached to this belt, she, pushing a stroller, periodically reached out and pulled the young boy closer as they walked and he strayed.

"Look," she said as they climbed aboard the moving walkway connecting the terminals, "It's a magic sidewalk."

For an instant, the short redheaded lad analyzed the metallic, moving, pathway, and — with some gentle guidance from his mother — hesitantly clamored on board. The young family stayed to the right so other, more hurried travelers, could pass.

"Him's my baby brother," the young man told everyone who walked past, pointing into the stroller. "His name is Lance."

The scurrying line of travelers, tugging rolling suitcases behind them as they dashed to planes, showed a variety of responses. "He's very handsome," said a smiling, matronly woman with a floral design carry-on. "That's nice," commented a dapper-dressed man in a pinstripe suit, carrying a computer case. Many simply smiled; others ignored the small lad.

When no one was in earshot, he studied Baby Lance, reaching into the stroller and rearranging the blankets of his infant brother.

"Him shouldn't be cold," he told his mom. "He could get sick."

She smiled and re-straightened the blankets, telling the young caregiver, "Thank you. You're a wonderful brother. You take very good care of Lance. Do you know I'm very proud of you?"

He hugged her leg. She patted his head. The walkway rolled on.

I was taken back to my own mother, who always reminded me of her pride in me, even in our last conversation. With her gone, it dawned on me that we don't hear, "I'm proud of you," so much as we get older.

We are quick to condemn our errors — and reticent to take pleasure in our accomplishments, mistakenly translating pride of accomplishment with arrogance, and self-satisfaction with conceit. In a desire to be modest or humble, we oft-times sacrifice the awe and wonder in what we accomplish for the frustration and irritation of what we do not. If I slip, I do not focus on my previous successes; rather I rebuke myself with hateful internal dialogue: "Wow, you blew it! What an idiot!" Our self-talk is sometimes so painful that it would be labeled abusive — and rightly so — if said to anyone else.

It is foolish to disregard one's flaws and ignore the lessons from our mistakes. Yet, I wonder what would happen if we more often told others — as well as ourselves — "I'm proud of you." It might not make a difference, but I cannot believe it would harm anything.

Fat on the inside

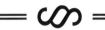

The most recent news from the diet world was too much for me to handle. Should you therefore be strolling the street and find small pieces of gray matter, be not alarmed for they are merely remnants of my brain, which hath exploded.

After decades of considering my ultimate goal to have the number stated on my driver's license be my honest-to-goodness weight — and actually achieving it — I have recently learned that one's weight is NOT the indicator of whether or not he is overweight. In case you didn't catch that, I shall repeat; not being overweight does not mean you are thin. (In fairness, it is my duty to warn you that this is the part that causes healthy brains to explode; tread warily.)

This revelation is based on a study yanked directly from Superman's Bizarro World. Dr. Jimmy Bell, a professor in London who was lead researcher, sums it up as such, "Being thin doesn't automatically mean you're not fat."

To me, one's weight NOT being an indicator of thinness is illogical; similar to, "having a full head of hair does not mean one is not bald." Or how about, "How much money one possesses has no relationship to one's wealth." Regrettably, in this brave new upside down skinny-is-fat world in which we find ourselves, 'tis true.

After conducting nearly 800 MRI scans to create "fat maps," which show where people store internal fat, Dr. Bell discovered people who maintain their weight through diet rather than exercise are likely to have major deposits of internal fat, even if outwardly slim. "The whole concept of being fat needs to be redefined," said Bell, who found that as many as 45 percent of women with normal BMI scores (a standard measurement of obesity) — and as many as 60 percent of men — had excessive levels of internal fat. The study refers to these individuals as "TOFIs": "thin outside, fat inside."

TOFIs existed even among professional models. Bell commented, "The thinner people are, the bigger the surprise." Yeah, I'd say that falls in the understatement department.

I picture a size zero super model strolling down the catwalk weighing a waif-like 79 pounds, able to be blown over by a sneeze. In the back room, Dr. Bell and company are making "fatty fatty two by four" jokes. Can you see how confusing this new reality can be?

If the scale is no longer the determinant of a healthy weight, I envision future health-conscious households having a room loaded with extensive equipment. In addition to a scale and exercise bike, I foresee a food scale, pedometer, stopwatch, BMI chart, body fat percentage calculator, portable MRI machine, hydrostatic weighing tank, DEXA machine (dual energy X-ray absorptiometry), calipers (for those emergency quick pinch tests), and a bioelectrical impedance scale.

Of course, after getting one's life in order to this level of detail, he or she will die of exhaustion. But then again, who knows? Maybe a future study will show that being dead isn't necessarily an indicator of failing health.

New diet pill – again!

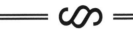

Alli, manufactured by GlaxoSmithKline, will be the first over-the-counter diet pill approved by the Food and Drug Administration, and soon graces the shelves of a drug store near you.

As those of us who diet reluctantly accept, there is no magic bullet for weight loss (sigh…). "People's hopes are ridiculously high when it comes to diet pills. That leads to disappointment and bad word of mouth," says an industry analyst. The VP of GlaxoSmithKline's weight control division points out, "We've done everything to go out of our way to be honest." They are trying to establish realistic expectations for this new entry into the diet market by providing a complete picture.

I say, "Kudos to them."

Let's take a closer look. In clinical trials, the FDA says people using Alli lost an additional two to three pounds for every five lost via diet and exercise. It does this by blocking the absorption of about one-quarter of consumed fat, which passes through the body, potentially resulting in loose stools. Moreover, about half the patients experienced side effects, including leakage and oily discharges.

Hmm, if that image doesn't make you want to eat less, what will?

In order to avoid these unpleasant effects, GlaxoSmithKline stresses keeping meals under 15 grams of fat. They even recommend starting the program when one has a few days off work, or, as an alternative, bring an extra pair of pants to the office.

I picture office cooler conversations:

"Hey, Scott, when you gonna start that new diet pill?"

"As soon as I can buy new pants."

"Wow! Positive attitude dude! Planning to lose so much weight and be skinny?"

"No, it's just, well, um, er, oh, never mind — read the label…"

Alli's "starter kit" includes a food journal, healthy eating guide and a fat and calorie reference. Its marketing exhibit features plates with sensible portion sizes, and a web site with an emphasis on diet and exercise.

The monthly cost of taking Alli, based on three times a day as suggested, will be between $60 and $75.

Let's recap shall we?

We have a pill with some relatively unpleasant potential repercussions. I mean, having to lug around an extra set of pants in the event of "side effects" seems a tad burdensome. I could be wrong; it could just be me.

More to the point, users consume less fat, record meals in a food journal, learn sensible portions, and exercise more. I sincerely applaud GlaxoSmithKline in devising a balanced, healthy weight loss approach.

However, will Alli sell? After all, if I'm eating less, tracking my food, lowering my fat, and increasing my activity, why do I need a pill?

Personally, I think I'll follow their lifestyle suggestions, skip the medicine, and use the $70 a month to buy some new pants — which I won't even need as a safeguard against side effects.

PAST MY TWENTIES

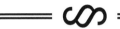

Recently, I had a revelation: I am no longer 22 years old.

There were obvious signs prior to this new dawning. For example, of late, in order to read small print, I must either remove my glasses or post the document across the room. Conversely, I must also use the "zoom" feature on my computer monitor to increase font size for virtually everything on screen.

I also must admit a tinge of guilt in continuing to list "brown" as my hair color on driver's license applications. Rather, "gray with a small bit of brown remaining" is more appropriate. (Since there is not enough space to use this accurate description, I rationalize "brown" as being as honest as possible.)

Oh yes, one other indicator that I am not 22 is that I am the biological father of a 23-year-old. Even the most forward thinking and mature 22-year-old would be hard pressed to have 23-year-old offspring.

Alas, despite this ever-growing chorus of facts, the dawning of my age did not fully appear until I weighed myself last week. I have been trying to knock off another six pounds and have stalled for some time. (OK, to be honest "some time" is approximately five years…) As I stood on the scale, glaring at the wretched red LED flashing between my toes in its hateful block numbers, a river of rushing thoughts coursed through me. In that cacophonous cascade of cognizance, one thought rose above all others: "I'm as diligent as I was 30 years ago but my weight won't budge. Back then; I lost three pounds a week! It's not fair!"

As I stomped from the scale (heading directly for the kitchen), a thunderbolt realization crashed through me: "It is not 30 years ago." No longer a young man of 22, I am now middle-aged. The rules for twenty-somethings do not apply.

Instead of trying to understand the ins and outs of a healthy weight and diet for a 52-year-old, I waste energy lamenting the fact that it is not as easy as it was "back then." How much precious time have I thrown away complaining about what no longer is rather than accepting the realities of what actually can be?

"I've never had to work so hard to lose weight." "I've always eaten this way." "I didn't have to work out when I was younger."

The thoughts and ideas we hold from earlier days were accurate and appropriate — in earlier days. But time moves forever backward into history, leaving us hostage to it, or empowered by the opportunities of the present.

This is neither a treatise against getting older nor a complaint about the travails of aging. Mostly — as long as my health holds out — I welcome the wisdom and peace of being an older man. But instead of grousing that I cannot lose weight like a 22-year old, it makes more sense to learn the rules for a 52-year-old — at least until I'm 53.

Drowning at 35,000 feet

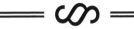

A healthy daily amount of water consumption is 48 ounces or more. Lately, I had been neglecting that requirement; the result being I was feeling a scooch "bulky." Therefore, be it resolved that while on my recent travels, I would drink eight glasses of water a day.

Whether in restaurants, at meetings, or on airplanes, I opted for the clear stuff. I am certain coffee and soda companies the country over were feeling a hit in their profits, but I felt proud for taking care of myself.

The downside about drinking so much water is the more one drinks; the more one's body needs to drink. After a short period of hydration, one's innards feel like desert sand if he goes a short time without water. The upshot is I began feeling antsy if I didn't have a water bottle within reach 24/7. Of course, another by-product of so much water is an excessive need to visit the rest room (or as I refer to it, "The Weight Reduction Cubicle").

With that as back-story, I boarded a three-hour flight to Houston.

Immediately upon reaching cruising altitude, I rose to use the lavatory, traversing the entire plane to get to its aft location. Upon returning, I recognized I was already thirsty and requested a new bottle of water, which did well to quench my thirst… and re-trigger the urge. Being near the front of the plane, each repetition of "the long walk," meant that I passed all the other passengers, leading me to feel self-conscious.

I was convinced they were whispering to seat mates, "What's up with this guy? You think he's got a thing about airplane bathrooms?"

Vanity and negative self-talk overruled by biology, I again un-clicked my seat belt and strode back to the lavatory, trying to avoid eye contact with the rows of flyers that had seen me parade the aisle twice moments earlier. The attendant smiled as if we were old friends, and opened the door for me as I approached.

Again, back to my seat, feeling parched. I resisted the urge for more refreshment, thinking if camels could traverse the vast expanses of dunes in North Africa, I could sit in a 737 for a couple of hours.

Sadly, I was mistaken. After repeating my "drink and release" pattern yet again, I was becoming intensely embarrassed and tried to sneak my way into the first class cabin for the next round, assuming upper crust folks would pay no heed to one of the riff-raff using their lavatory. The attendant gently pointed out, "for security purposes, main cabin passengers must use the facilities in the back of the plane," and steered me to this too-familiar landscape.

I wanted to counter her comment by asking how my small bladder could affect the safety of a 72,000-pound aircraft but in light of current airline security measures, decided against it.

As I walked yet again the long aisle, smiling awkwardly at the other passengers, I attempted to console myself with the thought, "at least I'm getting my exercise."

BY ANY OTHER NAME...

Words matter.

What we say to ourselves in our quiet spaces gives birth to actions. Life is the consequences of those events. If we wish to alter the course of our existence, to change its path, or to enjoy more the process, we must begin with the thoughts that steer it.

For example, let us take the overused, beaten down, threadbare expression: "I'm going on a diet." At the point when the peoples of all nations unite in solidarity and appoint me Head Honcho in charge of Global Linguistics, I shall ban the expression; I find its limited options lead to broken promises, loss of joy, low self esteem, and eventual failure.

In the stark and barren world where one "goes on a diet," it automatically implies one must — at some time — go off a diet. All is black and white; there is no gray; only "on" or "off," "good" or "bad," "following the diet" or "cheating." The gradations of in-between, which fill most of life, do not exist as, in that thought process, one cannot be "a little off" anymore than one can be "a little pregnant."

This perfect/awful thinking supposedly drives us to be perfect, which is an impossibility, so we inevitably label ourselves as "failures." Those of us who are recovering perfectionists know well the mantra of the dieter who has crossed to the dark side: "As long as

I blew it, I might as well really blow it! I can start again tomorrow." (or "Monday," or "next year"...) Once I have failed, I might as well get all of the "failing" out of my system, cleaning myself so I will be ready for to be perfect next time (ignoring the fact that it too will end up the same way).

Success in anything is rarely cut and dried. Rather the definition varies from one person to the next; sometimes even within oneself, depending on circumstances. Success is fluid; it requires parsing and nuance. More times than not, it is a two-step forward, one-step backward progression. In the sphere of success, one does not have it one day, lose it the next, regain it the third. She is more successful than she is not, learns from mistakes, makes adjustments — and therefore moves in a generally successful direction. Successful people have setbacks; the difference is they don't see them as the end of the line.

Only in mathematics and science, can lines can be clearly drawn. Two plus two will always equal four. In matters related of the heart and mind, crystal clear, straight-line delineation is not possible. We are not rigid robotroids fitting precision machined, pre-ordained molds. One cannot apply a formula to us and expect an exact result. We are too complex — and too human — for that.

The nice thing about that is if we accept that we will make mistakes, and can find a way to label them not as "failures," but rather "feedback," we can adjust, change, and even excel.

Words do matter; choose them wisely.

THE HUMAN TOUCH

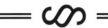

Since I was a boy, I have been fascinated by whiz-bang, LED-illuminated, state-of-the-art technology.

To mollify my inner child, I installed a home computer network and theater. My wife and I could actually talk about the groceries or pet care, but it's way cooler via email. Of course, I own a "smart-phone," one of those cellular devices that does everything (when it actually works). But, the pièce de résistance of my electronic empire is an all-encompassing, entirely programmable, tip-to-toe customizable, universal remote control — the Supreme Sultan of all apparatus electronic. Settled in the couch-throne, one can power up the television, adjust the surround sound, and commence the evening's entertainment with a twiddle of the thumb. All hail "Technology King!"

The irony is when all the electronic bloops and beeps cease, I resort to an extremely low-tech pastime to soothe me: I wander to a coffee house, order a cup of Joe, and peruse a newspaper. The tactile sensation of newsprint, coupled with the reverberation of others exchanging conversations at nearby tables, and the sensation of a warm mug in my hands, comforts me.

It's reassuring that still nothing replaces for me human closeness.

Recognizing me at the window table, the slightly overweight gentleman approached to introduce himself, "I read your column. I admire how you've maintained your weight. I wish I could be more like you."

Gratitude from people one does not know is exceptionally humbling, and I am always caught off guard. Yet, on that date, that particular morning, that moment in time, he was a gift.

Despite my apparent "victory" over obesity, the siren tug of late-night eating, super sized portions, and sugary treats does not fall deaf upon my ears. It is — even now, decades later — an unending battle. Neither smarter nor better than anyone else facing these demons, I am simply fortunate enough to have this platform to express what so many feel.

Stress still triggers me to eat (as does so much else) and the previous day had more than its share, so I camped in front of the refrigerator, until finally, at day's end, I forced myself to bed, angry and disgusted for having succumbed yet again. I berated myself, doubting my successes, ashamed of my weakness.

As an experienced veteran of these wars, I have learned to — despite sadness and resentment — quickly regain my footing and force myself into healthier behaviors as soon as possible.

That is the back-story that led me to this place; I was seeking to reclaim a sense of normalcy, something I felt I had destroyed the night previous.

He could not have known that, nor how encouraging were his comments. His alternate view of me helped more than he will ever know. If he is reading this, thank you. If my words inspired you half as much as you helped me, I am truly honored.

Sometimes, when one least expects it — but most requires it — you get what you need. Hang in there; we're in this together.

Difficult Until it Isn't

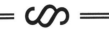

Despite contrary opinion, losing weight is not hard to do; it's amazingly simple:

- Eat a little less than you want
- Wait five minutes before you start
- Walk a little more than you would
- Focus on today (tomorrow will take care of itself)
- Repeat process until desired results are obtained

Voila! No pills. No bizarre food concoctions. No expensive plans. Simple. To the point. Successful.

As stated, it's not difficult.

Why then do Americans spend $33 billion a year on a process that can be outlined in fewer than 50 words? Here's the thing: Losing weight is not hard; changing one's mind to accept reality can be another issue.

I offer my own experience as case in point. I am no Johnny-Come-Lately to the rigors of dieting; having been on weight loss programs since before my memories were formed. As an overweight child who wore "husky" pants and XXL shirts, my mother served skim milk in (non-sugary) cereal and fruit for dessert. Doctors tried to shame me into losing weight; again and again forcing upon me those purple mimeographed pages overloaded with food lists, calorie counts, and dieting "secrets" (which never worked). Upon reaching adulthood, well-intentioned friends pointed out the health risks of obesity: heart disease, diabetes, and stroke; attempting to nudge me toward change. My life has been forged and melded in the furnace of dieting. I know this stuff better than the back of my slightly chubby hand.

So, why do I STILL have trouble sticking with it?

The answer? We make the process more difficult than necessary, gunking it up with all manner of artificial mental barriers and obstacles. Instead of accepting what must be done, I lament the process of change; stubbornly hanging on to the ineffective, seeking to finagle my way around what is required. I devise excuses for not waking in time to exercise. I tell myself, "just this once won't hurt" while nibbling leftovers from the refrigerator. I protest the higher price of healthier foods, opting in-stead for the long-term cost of greasy, crunchy, fried bags of chips.

Our thoughts are the problem, not the diets. We put ourselves at odds with our own best interest. At day's end, it is usual to want to "shut down," and unwind. Close the curtains. Turn off your mind. "Relax," coos the seductive call of well-worn behaviors, "You can start tomorrow."

"The price of freedom is eternal vigilance," said our third president. To obtain independence from the tyranny of destructive habits requires on-going diligent effort, as anything of value does. Yet, it is equally accurate — and too often forgotten — that when we pursue our passion, treat our bodies with respect, engage our better selves, and witness the results of those actions, there is no comparison to the elation, joyfulness, and euphoria that floods our soul.

At that point, the whole thing almost seems too easy.

INFECTED!

The *New England Journal of Medicine*, in a study of over 12,0000 people, suggests that obesity may be contagious, like a common cold. Apparently, when a study participant's friend became obese, that participant had a 57 percent greater chance of becoming obese himself. In pairs of close friends, one person becoming obese meant his friend had a 171 percent greater chance of following suit. "You are what you eat isn't the end of the story," summed up study co-author James Fowler. "You are what you and your friends eat."

As a child, if I insisted on going outside without a jacket, my mother warned, "If you get sick, don't complain to me." How will this new news play in today's health-conscious world?

"Mommy, can I play at Scott's house?"

"Isn't he the overweight boy down the street?"

"Yes, he's very nice. He's got cool toys."

"I don't think I want you to go there sweetie. You might catch a case of chubby."

"I won't mommy. Please."

"If you do, don't expect me to let out your seams."

I don't wish to poke fun, but can one be "infected" with obesity? The re-search, in my mind, simply points out the old adage, "Birds of a feather flock together."

As illustration, someone who enjoys triathlon training and a buddy who is an avid video game enthusiast might enjoy each other's personalities, and share similar views on politics and morality. Yet, would they hook up?

"Hey, Chris. Want to get together this weekend?"

"Sounds great. What shall we do?"

"We could grab something to eat, go to the mall. What do you think?"

"Sounds fun, but I've got my exercise regimen. How about we go to the pool first?"

"I can't swim."

"What about cycling?"

"Don't have a bike."

"We could go for a run."

"I'll just meet you there."

As Tevye said in Fiddler on the Roof, "A fish may love a bird. But where would they build a house?"

It is a function of human nature to feel best with people who are most like us and do as we do.

When I say, "you know?" I'm reassured when my friend says, 'Yeah, I do." That's why we're buds. If one enjoys sedentary, high-caloric activities, it stands to reason that so too will those around her. If she begins jogging, she didn't catch a dose of "fitness;" she changed a routine. Desiring to share that newfound interest, she will seek out others of similar mentality.

The biggest surprise to me was that this surprised them. Most people recognize that smoking and drinking are influenced by group standards, but apparently that realization is relatively new for obesity where so many still consider it a moral failing or merely a clinical condition. Obesity, like so much of life, is largely a function of behavior patterns. To change it, we must change what we do, not necessarily with whom we do it.

So — what the heck — try taking a walk with a friend. It couldn't hurt, and, who knows, you indeed might catch something: a healthy habit.

I AM NOT

I am Scott "Q" Marcus, whomever — or whatever — that is. Despite my belief that I think I know who I am, I admit to periodic doubt.

One thing of which I am certain however, is I am not a number.

Uncountable intertwined characteristics and traits make me "Me." On the simplest level, I am human, gender: male. I, with a couple billion of my closest friends, arrived on this small, ocean covered, awe-inspiring, nurturing planet via a chaotic and organized chain of events stretching so far back in time, that the very concept of that many millennia is beyond ability to imagine — even though I am gifted at imagining incredible things. I am a miracle of nature, a product of creation. I am: Life.

I am NOT a number.

I am a father and a husband. In our society, at this instant in history, those titles foster responsibilities ranging from the important: leaving a better world for our children (we're not performing well with that currently); to the mundane: I must shave every day (except weekends if my wife doesn't object).

I am a thinking, analytical soul. In my mind, I can articulate important concepts and — once in a while, when I'm very fortunate — even inspire others. Trillions of sparks criss-cross the synapses of my brain, flickers of my thoughts: the fate of the universe; the state of the nation; the choices on television.

I have philosophies, beliefs, and values. With those as guideposts, I have developed a road map that I presume (and pray) will lead me well to wherever is my final destination. From time to time I stumble and fall, to date always rising yet again. Therefore, I apparently must be determined, sometimes downright stubborn. Yet, I am also confused and wise, excited and bored, happy and sad, loving and lost, frightened and brave, teaching and taught, leader and follower, almost always — hopeful. All of these descriptors, words, and adjectives, are accurate in their portrayal of me, as are numerous others.

But I never describe myself via numerals. Neither does anyone else.

When friends greet me, they do not shake my hand, grasping warmly my shoulder, and say, "Hey 179, how are ya?" Instead, we hug, the warmth of his or her body held close to mine in a loving embrace. It is my name, not a number, spoken affectionately by someone about whom I deeply care.

They do not call to me by what shows on the morning scale.

I am not described as "179," "187", or — during particularly painful periods of my life — "250." My value, who I am, what I do, my legacy, does not fluctuate with the number of pounds reflected by what I ate nor by how many miles I jogged. That one number, my weight, although a description of a single, visible, component of WHAT I am, is virtually insignificant in the grand scale of WHO I am and what I am capable of accomplishing.

We are far more astounding than what any number, anywhere could ever make known.

Reclaiming her life

In line at the coffee house, she stood leaning on her left leg to prop up the baby on her hip. He sucked noisily on a yellow pacifier, watching over mom's shoulder as people queued behind her, huge blue eyes with an intense open stare greeting each new patron. The canopied stroller was therefore empty of its occupant. An SUV of child carrying conveyances, it was constructed to withstand the impact of an army of toddlers. Currently however, it served as transport, loaded with an assortment of quilted belongings, stuffed toys, a cell phone, bottles of baby food, and several zip lock bags distended with a plethora of toasted oats, wafers, and carrots.

On the opposite side of her infant son was her three-year-old daughter; clinging fiercely to mommy's leg for protection, burying her young face in her mom's thigh whenever anyone made eye contact. From her small hand, dragging across the tile floor was a white, weary, worn blanket, emblazoned with a smiling penguin.

Mom was only 32. Yet with her long dark hair hastily hoisted above her head in an elastic band, a gray oversized sweatshirt with "UCLA" (and numerous drool stains) across the front, and faded, fraying black sweat-pants, some days she felt as well worn as her attire.

She retained an attractive shape (albeit heavier from bearing two children), but could still "pretty up" quite nicely provided she had the time — or desire. She adored her husband; he was a kind, supportive, gentle man, who appreciated her for whom she was. Their financial situation required him to work long hours on the road, leaving her to attend to the house and the children. When he was in town, and the kids were finally in bed, and the maintenance of home chores at long last completed, romance ranked low compared to sleep. So neither of them spent as much time concerned about appearance as they had in earlier years.

Staying at home with her kids was vital, and she enjoyed it. It also provided her life with a value that working at the insurance company never could. Yet, everything bears a price. When you take care of everyone else, who takes care of you? The lack of self-attention was taking its toll and she felt it heavily.

She used to jog each morning; now she changed diapers, washed sheets, and prepared meals; always tasting while she cooked. In those all-too-fleeting, precious, rare moments of solitude, she escaped with a novel and a bag of chips. Every afternoon — just so she could get out — she scooped up the kids, walked to this place and ordered a cookie for them and a muffin for herself.

This afternoon, while the kids napped, she noticed her shape in the mirror and suddenly felt very old. In that instant came the spark of change. "Just take a step," she told herself. "Not everything, anything. It's a beginning."

When the clerk asked for her order, the whirlwind of thoughts collapsed into silence. She replied, "Juice, yogurt, non-fat milk, and a diet soda."

With that simple action, she felt alive again.

TAKING THE PLEDGE

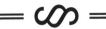

The pledge is all the thing; apparently, everyone's doing it.

Searching the Internet, I discovered 7,570,000 entries for "Take the Pledge." As examples, one can abandon old-fashioned round light bulbs in favor of newer CFL curly neon bulbs by taking the "Energy Star Pledge." According to their website, 549,033 bulbs have replaced! I'm a little concerned about that count however. For instance, if a bulb burns out, do they subtract one from the count?

Another organization requests we take an "End the Stroke Pledge." I can-not envisage anyone in favor of strokes, but question the necessity of having to swear allegiance publicly to ending them. Then again, I guess it cannot be harmful. Count me in.

One over-the-counter medicine asks us to pledge to create "germ-free defense zones" while also pledging to use their hand sanitizer. Personally, I think that's two pledges. It's also a little confusing; as illustration, am I in violation if I eradicate germs but use another product? I am not skilled in pledge-construction but do believe well worded pledges are devoid of loopholes.

A dedicated cluster of Macintosh computer users requests others not boot their computers into the Windows operating platform. I use a Macintosh. I didn't even know I could boot into Windows. Maybe I took that pledge without knowing.

I even stumbled across a group dedicated to improving our planet's atmosphere by asking cows to pledge to stop passing gas. How would one know if a cow made such a commitment; beyond that, who would be responsible for monitoring the contract? That would seem a rather unpleasant assignment.

So, in the interest of better dieting, I have devised — you guessed it — a pledge. Put down any tempting sweets, raise your right hand, and begin:

In the interest of better health, I (fill in your name) hereby pledge to...

- *Forgo all sugars and artificial sweeteners, eating only unprocessed, fresh, non-packaged foods*

- *Engage the services of a personal trainer who will ensure that I wake up three hours earlier, meditate extensively about better health, stretch extensively, and then finish with a 90 minute aerobic work out every day*

- *Record all food consumption in a food diary — but only after weighing it on a top-of-the-line electronic scale that computes fiber, fat, protein, sodium, and sugars*

- *Hire a top-end, live-in chef to ensure all food is prepared in the most healthful manner present nutritional science allows*

- *Read every food label, cross-referencing it with a portable food index that to be carried at all times, double-checking to make sure that I consume no trans-fats, very few calories, and a great deal of fiber (not being cows, we need not worry about fiber's side effects)*

- *Disregard the previous ridiculous commitments and make one small lasting change in my routine to eat a little less, walk a little more, and enjoy steady progress of a realistic program*

I BELIEVE

I believe there is more to each of us than we could ever know.

I believe there is one Source connecting everything, everywhere, always. It sits not on high, separate, watching passively, as we meander through the parade of choices composing our lives' stories. Instead it is inextricably intertwined within and around, nearer than our breath, no further than our thoughts.

I believe each and every thing we experience, feel, or think is born of that source. Every powerful spark of inspiration, tinge of emotion, or idea that will ever take shape is created of that place, centered deep within — and connecting — each of us. It is that innate connection we all share that has driven us from wanderers to farmers, thatched-leaf hut villages to expansive cities.

That force within us has guided us as we have fashioned astounding, spectacular, creations that can light the darkness, locate unseen illnesses, or further connect us: anywhere, anytime, with the tap of a SEND button. We hurl computerized, complex objects billions of miles across a darkened sky to land with pinpoint accuracy on far-flung worlds so distant that they are invisible to the naked eye — and would have remained unknown if not for others inspired to create by that exact same source we all share. We create because the Universe is in a constant state of creation. Being of it, we do the same.

We have founded treatments for afflictions and ailments from scurvy to smallpox, measles to polio. And someday, it is as sure as we exist that morning will dawn over a world devoid of cancer, AIDs, and Alzheimer's. We know we will find cures; we are merely in the process of bridging the distance between inspiration and implementation.

When we believe, we do spectacular, astounding things — and will do far more. It is what we do because it is who we are.

Our greatness has names, some known to many: Mother Theresa, Albert Einstein, Miguel Hidalgo, Fa-Ngoum, Martin Luther King, Jesus, Mohammed, and Buddha. Some are lesser known: you, the store clerk, the daycare worker, and me. Yet, within each is the precise unchanging power that created all who have come before and who will ever be.

Since we are part of the universe, we must be infused with the same stuff that created our rivers, mountains, oceans, and even our Mother Earth. Moreover, beyond that, the same universal force that envelops each of us, at all times, wherever we are, wraps the furthest star in the darkest night. Therefore, when we gaze far into the nighttime sky, we see some of our-selves. We cannot be separated from that which created us; it is denial of what we are, and what we can be.

I believe all this. And because I do, I am convinced that a force so powerful, so creative, so expansive to do all this, would never put anyone on this planet doomed to fail, whether her goal may be to change the future of millions or simply to lead a happier life for herself.

I felt we needed to be reminded. I sure do.

THE NEW ARRIVAL

It doesn't cry or use diapers, but rolls well and I can sit on it. OK, you guessed, I bought a new bicycle! I named it "Specialized Crossroads Sport" (it's easy to pick a name when it comes painted on it). It's a "comfort bike" because riding it is similar to riding a couch. (That is, if your couch rolls up hills and goes against the wind.)

Embarrassingly, by getting a new bike, I felt I was abandoning my old Schwinn Mesa. Of course, it didn't help when my wife said, "I can't believe you're retiring your old bike." Great, pangs of guilt; just what I needed! (Mental note to self: what does it say about me that I get emotionally attached to an inanimate object like a bike? Where is my therapist's phone number?)

First the back story: I'm not someone who does 100 mile cross country marathons, but I do find my way around town, utilizing my bicycle for commuting. I'll ride to meetings, drop off videos, or pick up some groceries. (If you go grocery shopping via bicycle, you save a heck of a lot of money also because you have to lug your goods on your back.) In essence, I do the usual "around town" errands on two wheels instead of four, saving me a few hundred dollars in gasoline, improving my health, and — as an added benefit — feeling I'm making a stand against Big Oil in some small manner.

A bicycle, just like a car (and us), requires regular looking after. Also as with a car, I am not able to provide said maintenance; so I take my metallic steed to the bike shop for adjustments. The last time I brought in my Schwinn, the "bike guy" said the whatchamacallit and the thingama-bob were wearing out.

"Not a big deal," adds he (easy to say if you're mechanically apt — unlike me), "But the cost to replace it is more than the bike is worth. You might want to consider one of the newer 'city bikes.'"

City Bikes, I discover, are for people like me; designed for short trips and tasks, they are more comfortable and do not make you stretch as much to reach the handlebars (a big deal, let me tell you). Infused with such newly acquired comprehension, I found my soon-to-be new best buddy at a local bike shop and plunked down my credit card.

After the exchange, it occurred to me:

- I spent almost $400 on a bike when I used to only buy $79 "specials."
- $400 on something I actually utilize beats the heck out of $79 on something I won't.

Formerly, I bought all manner of exercise paraphernalia that was eventually relegated to an expensive spot for hanging clothes I did not put away. Now, I know this bike will get oodles of use. Change has really occurred; slowly, over time, and without notice, like it usually does. But it's definitely here.

However, please join me in a moment of silence for my old bike. May he find a wonderful new home.

WATCH WHAT YOU SAY

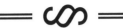

It never fails to astonish me what difference a few words can make. By the language we use, we can inspire others to feats of heroic sacrifice, create joyful laughter, or change the direction of our own lives. Words matter.

With that as backdrop, Alexander Kuzmin, the 33-year-old mayor of Megion, a Siberian oil town with a population of 54,000, has ordered his bureaucrats to stop using expressions such as "I don't know" and "I can't." If they refuse, they will be hearing a different phrase: "Find another job." In a world of customer service representatives who would rather point fingers than solve problems, you've just got to love this guy!

Kuzmin has banned these and 25 other expressions as a way to make his administration more efficient. Some of the other prohibited phrases are "It's not my job," "It's impossible," "I'm having lunch," and "There is no money." To reinforce the prohibition, a framed list of the banned expressions hangs on the wall next to his office.

"Before," says one staff member, "It was so easy to say 'I don't know.' Now before reporting to the mayor we prepare several proposals on how the problem can be solved."

Isn't that something? By being forced to avoid certain words, people accomplish more — or at least come up with alternatives.

When you analyze it, it makes great sense. After all, we think in words. Sure, we're creative sorts; but the process by which we translate those flashes of intuitive brilliance into action is via the internal conversation ever present in our minds. The repetition of that exchange, over years, shapes our view of ourselves, how we re-act to outside events, and there-fore the actions that become our lives. If one wants to permanently change the construction of his life, he must start with the building blocks: those internal words, thoughts.

Take for example the common belief, "I can't lose weight." If you, like, are forever fighting gaining weight, try this: Instead of saying "I can't lose weight," say out loud with conviction, "I can lose weight. I just don't want to go through all the work it will take." You will no-tice — virtually immediately — an uncomfortable feeling welling up inside you. Why? Words, thoughts, feelings, and beliefs are bound together tighter than a psychological Gordian knot. Disconnecting them is impossible.

I create my beliefs; I do so to make my life run smoother. If I repeat, "I can't" enough times, I am absolved of the responsibility of trying, leaving time for other "more realistic" pursuits. If I change "I can't" to, "I won't," I am forced — at least in my internal dialogue — to jus-tify my motives, which can sometimes feel rather "messy." It's much easier to sidestep the responsibility; after all I'm already very busy.

When I say something different, I feel something different. Different emotions elicit different thoughts. New actions come from such un-tried thoughts. Life is the result of actions.

Say something different. Repeat often. Watch for new results.

TRYING TIMES

I am trying to lose a few pounds (again).

I'd put odds on the fact that I'm not the only person in our sleepy burg with such a stated goal. Others are trying things too: stop smoking, be more active, spend more time with their families. As a whole, we TRY many things. The more important question is, "Are we DOING them?"

I wish I could remember which wise sage pointed out "trying" is "saying 'no' with grace."

A friend lost into your past surprises you by reappearing while you are squeezing cantaloupes at the grocery store. Pre-ordained ceremonial niceties commence, "How are your kids? What's your husband doing these days? Are you still working at the same place?" It's a pleasurable oasis of exchange with someone who used to be close. Yet, after the first few paragraphs, what remains to be said? An awkward silence slithers between you until finally you utter, "Let's get together and catch up. It's been too long."

She replies warmly, "I'll try and call you next week, OK?"

"Sounds great," you say before exchanging air kisses, and continuing on your mission of securing the finest produce. You know she won't call. You know you won't either.

She could have said, "No, I'm too busy," or "No, I'm not interested." Rather than such bluntness, she replies with the socially approved, milquetoast, "I'll try."

Underlying her intentions was, "No" — delivered with grace.

In those situations, "I'll try" is caring; it diffuses rough, confrontational, unkind exchanges. However, in so many other circumstances, we use "try" as a justification for our own unwillingness to change. After all, what if we give up or decide later that the objective takes too much effort? It hurts to boldly state, "I AM losing a few pounds," only to face questions at a later time when well-meaning friends inquire, "How's the diet going?" It saves face to be able to reply, "I tried, It didn't work," rather than, "I wasn't willing to do it," or "I changed my mind."

In reality, what is there to "try?" Am I actually eating less? Am I really more active? Select one: "yes" or "no." If I choose to not act on my own words, I am not "trying," I am simply "not doing."

Of late, I find myself stating proudly to anyone within earshot what I am "trying" to do. In actuality, I am setting the stage for the excuses I might use at another time.

"I am trying to lose weight," I say.

My friends nod in agreement, commiserating. "It's tough, isn't it?"

"Yes. But I'm really trying hard."

"Good for you," they say, "I admire you."

Yet, my scale has not moved; my waistline has not shrunk. The glaring unavoidable reality is I am not "trying," I am stagnating. The moment has arrived; it is time to stop "trying" and begin "doing."

The use of the word "try" is so addictive; it's tough to ratchet up the commitment to "I'm doing." But I'm trying.

No one does that

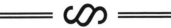

"Howdy bud. Welcome to the Comerite Inn. Where ya from?"

"Northern California," I say, dropping my bags on the lobby floor.

"California, huh? I've never been there. Anyway, consider this your home for a few days."

"Thanks. I'm just glad to be on solid ground."

While I fill out the registration form, he references the hotel's amenities, "Breakfast is served from six to nine. Ice is next to the elevator. And every room comes with free wi-fi."

"Before I go to my room, could you point me to a restaurant within walking distance? I'd like to get something light before it gets too late."

"Save your feet; the hotel shuttle can take you; no charge."

"No thanks, after sitting all day, I could use the walk."

Confused, but caring and concerned, he replies, "Really? Walk? It's at least a quarter mile to the closest restaurant."

"Oh, I didn't realize that."

"Yep, that's why I suggested the van."

"I didn't mean that," I clarify "I'd prefer a longer walk. Anything about a mile down the road?"

Inspecting me as if I just said, "I like stabbing sharp objects in my eyes," he continues, "A mile? You sure you don't want me to call the driver?"

"No, just the directions."

"Partner, nobody walks around these parts. It's just not done."

"So if you're dieting, or just want to get exercise, what do you do?"

He references his large belly, overhanging his belt and pants by several inches, "Do I look like someone dieting who 'gets exercise?'"

"Oops, sorry. However, I'd still like to walk."

"To be honest, I don't know how to walk there because it's all highway. If you had a car, I'd say take I-35 about a mile. Turn right. You'll see Rosi-ta's."

"So, why can't I just walk?"

"I wouldn't recommend anyone walk the interstate, too dangerous."

"What about the frontage road? I don't need to go on the freeway."

"No sidewalks." He points to the street.

"I see. So what do you do if you just need to go a couple of blocks?"

"I told you; hop in the SUV. This city's built for tires, not feet. Let me see if Shelly knows a way to walk there."

Calling out to the stockroom behind the registration desk, he bellows, "Hey, Shel; a guest wants to walk to Rosita's. How would he do that?"

From behind the wall, a woman's voice responds, "Walk? Huh? Doesn't he know there's a shuttle?"

"Yep, still wants to walk."

"Did you tell him it's free?"

"Sure did, I think it's a 'California thing.'" He smiles at me. I nod knowingly.

"Can't do it, he'd be road kill," she calls, "shuttle's his only option — un-less he wants to eat upstairs."

He looks back at me, shrugging his shoulders. "Might as well just use our restaurant. Save yourself the hassle. Safer too."

Accepting the inevitable, I nod, "Where's your restaurant?"

"Second floor. Take the elevator on the right."

"Can you point me to the stairs?"

"Stairs, are you kidding?"

LUCKY 13

As a 17-year-old, I dropped almost 100 pounds, becoming thin for the first time in my life. By 22, I regained most of it. During that period, I avoided attending meetings, which had worked so well, and therefore suffered the consequences. Funny, isn't it? You'll do everything you can — except the one thing that gets you the results you want. Contrary creatures, we humans can be.

Finally returning, I sat in a meeting, embarrassed, ashamed, and sad; a thin, middle age woman addressed the assemblage. "My name's Betty," she said, holding up her "before photo," "I've maintained a 100 pound weight loss for ten years."

"One hundred pounds," I thought. "I couldn't even do that for half that time; no way I'll make it." It seemed the impossible dream.

This week, I am celebrating 13 years at my correct weight, after losing 70 pounds. (I had not regained everything I lost in earlier years; some lessons do stick.)

In these 4,700 plus days since I achieved "goal weight," I've learned much. Space doesn't allow for everything, yet, there's room for a few observations; provided in the interest of helping others achieve the success I have been fortunate enough to experience.

- Losing weight is not linear; it's four pounds down, two pounds up; losing five, gaining three; dropping one and flat lining for a month. It's up and down with (hopefully) more downs than ups.

- The internal "battle" about food choices does not cease. Speaking for myself, I merely have become more accustomed to the ongoing drone of the voices jostling for position in my head; now choosing to listen to the positive, healthful ones more often than the others. As for attitude: I've learned to quiet the inner jerk that wants to berate me for my slip-ups, of which there are still plenty. After all, if shame was motivational, I would never gain a pound.

- Getting to one's correct weight is not a panacea for all life's ills. My kids still do things I dislike. My wife and I still sometimes are at loggerheads. And yes, I continue to be frustrated with the world. But since I'm happier, I handle these issues better.

- Dieting "success" makes one no better a person. Weight does not determine moral value, and I am therefore not superior because of what my scale reflects. I am happier — because I beat back a demon that ran my life for too many years, NOT because of what I weigh.

Lastly and strangely, having a weight problem has emerged as my greatest blessing. I used to curse my life, but if not for the work I had to do to change, I might never have developed my love for life, the great relationships I now share, nor would I have had the honor of writing this column. Sure, these might have developed from a different path. But I didn't take — or wasn't given — that option. It doesn't matter; I cannot change what was not.

The fact is I am where I am, and more importantly, pleased to be here. That's worth waking up for.

CURING WHAT DOESN'T AIL

Question: Why is dieting replete with unsubstantiated claims, transparent falsehoods, and blatant aggrandizements that we would never accept elsewhere? No way we would believe — even in 300-point screaming fonts: "NEVER FILL YOUR GAS TANK: DRIVE FOREVER!" or "FLY ANYWHERE WITHOUT BOARDING A PLANE!" So, why oh why, does the weight loss amphitheater attract so many charlatans? More important, why do we continue to pony up our money and dreams to invite them back?

I am prompted (or pushed) into this tirade by yet another ad with still one more banner headline touting "the next amazing discovery" to lose weight without adding exercise or changing diet. This particular magical cure-all comes in the form of a supplement preventing hunger pangs, therefore causing one to eat less, ultimately losing weight. Extensive writing described the methodology and research leading to the enchanted formula. The first thing I observed, being a natural skeptic of such promises, is the copy had no fewer than 15 asterisks referencing four-point type stating "these statements have not been evaluated by the (FDA)." My translation: Results cannot be proven.

OK, for the sake of argument, I am aware that next-generation discoveries take time to withstand the rigors of the scientific method; and it's possible — even likely — that valuable life-enhancing tools can perform prior to receiving government's stamp of approval.

So, let's go beyond that. The basic seductiveness all these products share is that their claims, at first blush, do seem to make sense: No hunger equates with less eating. Less eating means less of me. Sounds accurate, yes? Yet, not everything that appears logical on the surface withstands intellectual scrutiny. As illustration, it seems to make sense that if one glues feathers to his arms and flaps hard enough, he should lift off. What both premises lack is grounding in reality.

Being obese most of my life, having only tilted the scales at my correct weight for 25 percent of my five-plus decades, I understand dieters. Moreover, I work with, coach, and speak to thousands of kindred spirits every year. The bottom line? Not ONE person is overweight because he suffers from hunger pangs! None. Nada. Zip. We — people battling weight — just don't get hungry. Why? Because we're eating too much when we're NOT hungry; therein lies the true problem. When you're gobbling a box of chocolate cookies, a brick of cheese, and bag of chips, HUNGER is not the driving force; it's not even in view.

Skinny people eat from hunger (physical need for food); overweight folks respond to appetite (emotional and external drives to eat). Should this "unevaluated" supplement even be successful at removing hunger, the problem would still persist. Unless it can remove the emotional forces driving over-consumption, it's as useless as a sugar pill.

One's thoughts, emotions, and beliefs about eating — or anything — cannot be changed via supplement, medicine, or herbal concoction. Rather, that only occurs through increased consciousness, perseverance, and a patient, nurturing, sense of self-control. When we can harness those in pill form, I'm first in line at the pharmacy.

FOR WANT OF A NAIL

As the proverb goes, the knight had no nail to attach the horseshoe to the hoof of his trusty steed. As a result, unable to ride to the castle to alert the army of the approaching enemy, the fortress fell, the king was captured. The kingdom collapsed.

For want of a nail, a kingdom was lost. Small actions can have enormous consequences.

Recently, it became apparent that I was becoming entirely too friendly with the assortment of bread products in our kitchen. When bored, frustrated, depressed, lonely (insert feeling), I wandered to the pantry and mindlessly consumed a few English muffins, medicating away whatever messy emotion I had at the moment: Ta-da, denial via breadstuffs!

The prime rule of the universe portends, to do what you've always done will get you what you've always got. Try as we might to ignore this edict, results remain unaltered. Add to that sobering observation the reality that my waistline had been stubbornly refusing to shrink, and, alas, the impetus fell solidly on me — and my bulging midsection — to modify my behaviors, or remain on the current path of frustration.

In what to me seemed a feat of superhuman strength, via a heated internal conversation in front of the bakery section at my local grocery store, I forced myself to forgo my weekly ration of English muffins and hamburger buns, a minor victory for some, but requiring for me enormous will-power. Concerned I might starve in the next seven days; I loaded my shopping cart with healthier alternatives, bushels of vegetables. I might go gently into the carbless night, but I shall venture forth well stocked.

What transpired because of this small act was that each time I wandered mindlessly to the now-bare pantry, I was confronted with empty shelves, forcing me to engage in alternative behaviors. Late night eating, always a rough spot, lost much of its "fun factor" without my comfort foods. After all, eating lettuce at 11PM? Why bother? Might as well suck on Styrofoam, so I plopped into bed earlier.

More sleep begat more energy, as well as a diminished drive for post-sunset calorie consumption. Furthermore, the muffin's "companion foods," burgers, cheese, spreads; no longer had a buddy. They remained isolated and uneaten in the refrigerator. The result? In addition to lower grocery bills, my weight is dropping at a slow, albeit regular, pace.

But isn't that the way it goes? We convince ourselves that change re-quires massive adjustments and alterations, a Herculean effort. Having fully stocked lives and faced with the prospect of a massive rebuilding of all our patterns, we opt to remain mired in the sticky goop of stagnation. Once no longer able to shoulder the dissatisfaction, we timidly remove one miniscule temptation, unaware that by removing that particular plank from the wall, a cascade of others follows, revealing vistas we could not imagine.

One insignificant step, one seemingly incidental change, causes a domino effect, affecting levels unforeseen. We cannot know the outcome of every action; yet we can still pound in one, tiny, nail.

APPROPRIATE DIET ATTIRE

Dieters, at least those of us that would consider ourselves "professionals," have standard rituals revolving around weighing ourselves. Most will not stand on a scale until they've visited the rest room. Without being indiscreet, when one thinks about why that behavior is a prerequisite to measuring your weight, the reason becomes obvious; make sure you have shed every last possible ounce before weighing in. After all, the coffee you drank last hour weighs almost a pound, whether located in a cup or in you. You don't want to weigh with it. Therefore, in the name of accuracy, we refer to rest rooms as "weight reduction cubicles." Only the brave, foolish, or untrained don't make that pit stop prior to approaching the scale.

There are other methods to shed last minute poundage. Removing accessories and shoes are common. I understand the need to take off hiking boots or work shoes. However, on more than one occasion, I've seen people remove socks and rings. Please understand they are not obsessing over a few ounces, merely dedicated souls seeking the utmost precision. Accurate record keeping depends on detail.

I am amazed by how much "stuff" men carry. Not having a purse to lug about one's belongings is not a disadvantage to an ingenious gentleman. A handful of change, several keys, and a wallet are common. Beyond that, out come pens, pencils, small tools, magnifying glasses, and glass cases from shirt pockets. From one's pants, he will pull a cell phone, wallet, money clip, and several dollars in change. Finally in addition to removing their belts, a great number carry a knife or all-purpose utility tool. I am amazed there are not more workman's compensation claims for back-aches by the sheer mass most guys carry attached to their bodies.

Many times, a dieter trying to drop "those last few ounces" by disrobing further than I feel comfortable has turned me a shade of crimson. To illustrate, a woman three ounces above her desired weight had completed all the standard ploys; all to no avail. She was considering her options while I waited.

Jokingly, I said, "Too bad they have laws about nudity, huh? Those clothes are holding you back."

She replied. "Can you look away?"

Taken aback, I said, "Uh, how will I see the scale?"

"I'm not taking off my clothes. You can turn around again in a moment."

I faced away, giving her the privacy she requested. From the corner of my eye, I saw her arm disappear inside her sleeve, heard rustling fabric, and from the same sleeve, an offending garment, her brassiere, clenched in her fist, came back out. She placed it on the counter and said, "OK, weigh me now."

Being male, I was flummoxed. I cannot take off my socks without removing my shoes. How could she remove an undergarment without taking off her outer clothes? Figuring out such mysteries is not my job however, so I refocused my attention on the scale.

"You made it. Congratulations," I said, recording the number in her booklet.

She smiled, collected her belongings and responded, "I'm glad I used an underwire. The other one might not have weighed as much."

Benefits

So say marketing gurus: "People don't buy what they need; they buy what they want." In common language that means the majority of decisions (whether buying a product or into an idea) are based on feelings before fact. That's not to say we're irrational; it is to admit that emotion puts the key in the engine and turns it on, logic steers.

To lock in this concept, countless people NEED to stop smoking; virtually each one would agree. Why don't they do it? They don't WANT to. There are folks who NEED to get out of bad relationships, find new jobs, and rearrange unhealthy lifestyles. Why don't they do it? Again, they don't WANT to.

And prior to going on a diet, I — as every other obese person on the planet — desperately NEEDED to lose weight. Even though I suffered brutal chest pains, felt my life was out of control, and my self-esteem was non-existent; I still possessed unlimited excuses about why I couldn't go on a diet. The genuine reason was I simply didn't WANT to. Plain. Simple. To the point.

We start WANTING to change when we focus on what we will get from the process of change, "benefits" as they are referred to in sales lingo. What propelled me was when I accepted that my marriage was failing. Upon that realization; it occurred to me I might end up lonely if I didn't do some personal remodeling. Suddenly, I very much WANTED to transform, to be attractive. (Truth be told, if women considered a 250-pound, 44-inch, flabby, middle age man with low esteem, backaches and chest pains to be a "catch," I might never have lost the weight.)

I needed to change for years; yet remained stagnant. The instant I wanted to, I began. Want to inspire someone, including you? Speak to the emotions before the intellect; you'll be ahead every time.

Contrary beings, we humans can be, so even though we start seeking happiness, control, energy, attractiveness, flexibility, self-esteem, pride, or a longer life (among others); we lose sight of the benefits and begin paying attention only on the figure illuminated on the scale. That numeral is simply a reflection, a short-lived snapshot; one miniscule, trivial segment in a vast, expansive, exhilarating landscape of all that's shifting. Yet like an addicted gambler betting the farm on one throw of the dice; if the number goes down, we're in like Flint, exhilarated and prepared to move forward. Should its pronouncement be unwanted, we give up, sacrificing the whole host of joyful benefits waiting down the road. We're in or we're out; there is no middle ground.

How marvelous would it be if we could measure ALL the reshaping taking place during this journey? Beyond pounds, we could count attitude, self-esteem, pride, joie de vivre…

It requires confidence, a deeper understanding of oneself, patience, and commitment to focus on the cornucopia of stimulating internal changes coming forth in the process. Ironically, they are some of the principal benefits received from all that hard work. Each time we do that, it's proof the process is working.

GIVING THANKS IN TOUGH TIMES

"May you live in fascinating times" is an old curse; the logic being if one chronicles history, "fascinating times" were jam-packed with upheaval. Turbulent, troublesome, frightening, epoch-making periods; anyone experiencing them would be upset, frightened, and anxious.

I point this out because, with the way the world is, one might make a case that we are currently experiencing "fascinating times," and that future historians will find the initial piece of the 21st century to be chock-full of tumult, worthy of study for generations yet to come. For them, that may be well and good, yet for us in the present, I don't think I stand alone when I pray we figure out soon how to get along a little better.

Giving thanks in such chaotic times is not simple. It feels difficult and trivial to find positives when all around seems urgent. However, to do so, requires a refocus on what one has, rather than a sadness of the way it is not. Saying "Thank you," lightens the heart, and loosens life's burdens — if only for a moment, making living worthwhile. Now, more than ever, it is essential to express gratitude for what one has. We are still blessed in many ways.

I can be thankful to sit at a table with family and friends, sharing food, conversation, and stories. We will laugh at where we have been, even if we disagree about where we are headed. We are not a perfect family unit; but we are what we are. I give thanks, and send a prayer to those less well off.

I am grateful to live where I do. Sure, I complain about excess rain and a hidden sun. I lament the dreary fog in the morning, and the wind in the afternoon. Yet, on the grand perspective, this patch of Mother Earth is no less than stunning. Endless forests of trees on majestic mountains caress the heavens; rushing, raging, rivers cut through strong stone canyons in their never ending race to become part of a breathtaking vista of world's greatest ocean. I reside in a postcard photograph; is that cool or what?

Contrary to how I was raised, I taught my children, "Do what you love, the money will follow." Although it took me four decades to heed my own advice, it has worked out and I am uplifted by what I do. While others never leave a squalid village, and have no hope, I have traveled far, seen much, and spoken to many. I am again grateful.

I am not alone, residing in a community, a true enclave of people who greet me with handshakes and "hellos." We still ask about each other's children. We share personal successes and setbacks. I have no interest in living elsewhere; I am gratified to be where I am.

My story is different than yours; each of us travels his own path. However, it is my purest intent that in my appreciation, I kindle within you a smile or joyful thought that you will share with others, lightening your day and theirs.

Saying thank you might not change a life. However, it sure won't hurt.

GETTING THROUGH THE HOLIDAYS

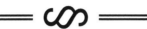

When I first starting writing this column, I decided to focus on the thoughts, feelings, and beliefs required to lose weight. That doesn't preclude me providing some practical advice now and then. Since the holidays are one of the more difficult times, it seemed appropriate to offer a few suggestions that have (usually) guided me safely through this time of year. You will not find a collection of low-fat recipes or traditional diet tips forthwith; I leave those to others who excel in that arena. Instead, I hope these few thoughts and ideas triggers inspiration on how to help your diet survive the remainder of the year.

- **Set realistic expectations**
  Losing weight during December is unlike other months. That's not an excuse to consume an entire pecan pie or two pounds of Hanukkah Gelt; but don't expect to find it as easy as it is other times of the year. (Of course, I'm not sure it's ever "easy" but you get my drift, right?) Be gentle on yourself if you slip up, just don't give up.

- **Realize the holidays are not every day of December**
  In reality, there are only about seven to ten troublesome days during November and December. Although that may be more concentrated than other periods, it still leaves a lot of time to maintain control. On a calendar, mark down the

days that will be the most difficult, including travel and visitors. Once you actually see the tough times, it relieves some of the stress and allows you to plan better for those periods.

- **THINK. THINK. THINK.**
Excessive eating is a habit, a pattern of activity done without thinking. To weaken a habit, one must therefore slow down and engage brain cells. How? Wait ten minutes before eating. If, at the end of that period, you still feel the urge, have ONE. Repeat the waiting cycle before getting seconds. Most people find they get busy during the delay and forget the temptation. It might not stop excesses, but delaying what you consume still helps reduce calories over the long haul.

- **Realize no one is overweight "because of the holidays"**
We tend to think that we'd be thinner if it weren't for the indulgences of the holidays. Reality check: If the only time overweight people ate excessively was during holidays, we wouldn't be overweight. Assuming we indulge at every celebration (including those such as Flag Day and Admissions Day) we're still only counting about 30 days a year, less than ten percent of the time. The holidays don't throw us off; it's all that time in between holidays where we continue on our eating sprees. We say, "Well, as long as I blew it, I might as well start again when the holidays are over."

I don't mean to burst a bubble, but the holidays — at least those around this time of year — have been in existence for a few thousand years. They are not stopping anytime soon. However, with some fore-thought and focus, one can stop the yearly weight cycle and really have something healthy to celebrate in January.

Red wine dieting

People send me things.

After one of my columns which portrayed a middle-aged woman inspecting her-self in the bedroom mirror while her husband lovingly observed, I received a card from an 83-year-old woman who said that after 65 years of marriage, her husband still looks at her "that way" and she loves it. You go elderly couple! You inspire me.

I wrote about riding my bike. Someone called me and said she knew Lance Armstrong, and would send him that column. That's kind of cool — to think that Lance Armstrong would read my words. I like to think it was what inspired him to win the last Tour de France. (Of course, I like to think I inspired Michelangelo's statue of David also. The odds are about the same.)

I receive a great deal of email about what I write. Embedded in the bits and bytes of electronic communication that I download to my trusty Macintosh are questions about weight loss, motivational observations about change, poems with a dieting theme, and references to stories on the web.

One such hyperlink terminated in an article on MSNBC.com entitled, "Big Fat Does of Red Wine Extract Help Obese Mice Stay Happy, Healthy, and Live Longer." (On the internet, they are apparently not limited to short headlines.) The gist of the article (which later made national news) was that a study by the Harvard Medical School and the National Institute on Aging showed that an ingredient in red wine, resveratrol, lowers the rate of diabetes, liver problems, and other "fat-related" ill effects in obese mice. Fat-related deaths even dropped 31 percent when mice were given a supplement derived from resveratrol.

The mice did not have to change what they eat, rather they were kept on a high-calorie diet, which one scientist called a "McDonald's Diet." Not only were they about as healthy as normal mice, but they were as agile and active as their lean counterparts when it came to exercise. Said the doctor, "They're chubby but inside they look great."

I ponder future repercussions on humans. Could it be that in upcoming decades the concept of healthy dieting undergoes a complete transformation? In the present, I choose salads, high-fiber unprocessed grains, and lean protein — while making sure I walk or ride my bike regularly. Is it conceivable that years from now — while in a constant haze of red wine-induced inebriation — I find myself gorging on a cholesterol feast of dripping chili cheese burgers on double thick buns, extra cart loads of French fries, gooey chocolate sundaes, and peanut butter chocolate candies?

When approached by a well-intentioned (but uneducated) stranger distressed about my 82-inch waist, I reply, "Thank you for the concern but I'm in training for a marathon."

BABY STEPS

I'm Jacob. My parents call me "big boy" even though I don't wear big boy pants like Ryan. But he's almost three; I've got two years until then.

Mommy, Daddy, Ryan, Buster, and I live in a big house, although Buster has to go outside to do his business. I don't know what kind of business a dog would have; I don't think it's like Daddy's, because no one makes Daddy go outside to do his business; he just drives there.

I'm learning a lot, like how to walk. Daddy likes to hold both my hands way up above my head and guide my feet. First left, then right; back and forth. Sometimes, he pulls too high and my feet don't touch the ground. I want to cry because it hurts my arms, but I don't want Daddy to feel bad. He's doing the best he can.

I want to walk by myself; it's time, but it's scary.

In our living room, we have a coffee table. Why it's called that, I don't know; they drink coffee in the kitchen — more to learn. Anyway, I pull myself up along the edge of that table, hang on to the sides and walk around and around it. I feel powerful when everyone has to move their feet to let me pass.

Today, I decided not to hold on. Putting both hands forward in case I lost my balance, I slowly let go. I was wobbly, but you would be too with a big wad of diaper between your legs. It was so exciting; it caused me to drool all over my shirt! Mommy laughed and said, "You can do it big boy!" Daddy got the camera; he takes pictures of everything. If he ever shows those naked pictures of me, I'll be upset.

I only walked four steps before I fell; I was so upset with myself. Everyone else walks all over, they even run and skip. I couldn't make it across one room. "What a dummy!" I thought, and was sure my family was em-barrassed by me.

But that's not how they saw it, what a reaction! Mommy hugged me so tightly I couldn't breathe. "You're my big boy!" she said. Daddy did a high five with me, "Way to go little man!" he laughed. Buster barked. Ryan clapped. So did I. We all giggled. Wow! Trying new things is really excit-ing!

I can't wait to grow up. By how they treated me, I know that when you grow up, you don't abuse yourself for your mistakes; you just pick your-self up and move forward. Because, to be honest, if they would have called me "stupid," or insulted me for not succeeding, I don't think I would have tried again. But I did — and made seven steps!

Grown ups are always so kind in what they say, forever supportive and encouraging, just one happy notion after another. It must be wonderful to live in such empowering thoughts; why would anyone not do that?

My first adult lesson: Speak kindly to yourself for trying, not insult your-self for falling. It keeps you moving forward.

Ooops, gotta go. I think I need a new diaper.

Easy as pie

∞

"Are you going to finish eating that?"

"I want to give it a few minutes to see how I feel. I'm not sure I'm full."

"It sure looks tasty."

"Yes, you're right. It does look tasty. As a matter of fact, it is extremely tasty."

"You know, I love that kind of pie."

"Thank you for sharing. Most folks do."

"If you decide you don't want it, I'd be glad to polish it off it for you."

"What a surprise. I'll make a note so I don't forget."

"How long will it take to determine whether you're full or not?"

"What's with all the questions? Are you taking a survey? Do you have a pending appointment and need to take a piece of pie with you?"

"No, it's just that it would be a real shame to throw it away. I don't want it to go to waste."

"It would be more of a shame to waist it — if you catch my drift."

"Yeah, cute. It's just a small piece. It's not like eating the whole thing."

"You're right. Except I already had a slice so I'm trying to focus on the whole picture. When I eat without thinking, I regret it later, so trying to slow down and appreciate my food, not just shove it down. It's kind of a 'quality versus quantity' thing. If I weigh my options, I don't have to weigh myself."

"If you want my opinion, it's not a life-changing decision like buying a house that will cost you hundreds of thousands of dollars. It's a silly sliver of pie for goodness sake."

"And your point is?"

"No need to stress out about it."

"I am not stressing. I'm thinking, analyzing, even pondering. But since you brought up money, this is similar to having a bank account, but instead of dollars, I have calories; I can spend them anyway I want, but if I spend too many, I end up in debt. I used to spend myself into bankruptcy. I don't like that feeling. I'm trying to change."

"Couldn't you take out a calorie advance loan and repay it tomorrow?"

"Been there, done that; I'm in caloric debt for the entire year. I've got to start paying it back soon, stop telling myself, 'you can begin tomorrow;' the hardest thing is getting started. If you could give me some quiet, I'd appreciate it."

"Should I go somewhere else?"

"Is that possible? Can inner voices do that?"

"I'll tell you what, just let me have this one final piece and I promise I'll shut up and never bother you again."

"You say that every time."

No more potato salad

Each dieter does it differently. Some eat a lot but look forward to exercise to burn it off. To me, looking forward to exercise is akin to eager anticipation of a root canal. Ain't gonna happen.

My method of staying on track is by removing temptation; i.e., if it's not here, I won't eat it. Should you inspect my refrigerator, you would lay view to a vast amount of empty space. It's a Spartan existence, but — for the most part — it works.

My mother used neither exercise nor my "minimalist" approach. Rather, she simply controlled her portions. Wow! What a novel concept: Eat well and eat the correct amount. Who would have thought?

Yet, therein lies a rub.

Whenever I visited, she would organize some form of get-together "in Scott's honor." Aunts and cousins would converge on Saturday afternoon to see how the Northern California component of the clan was surviving. Hugs. Conversation. Photographs. And of course, food. Lots and lots of food.

Across numerous tables would span a landscape of desserts, rolls, cheese, desserts, cold cuts, desserts, drinks, and — did I say — desserts. If ten people were expected, we had foodstuff for 50. "Food shortage" was not in her vocabulary.

For Mom, being encircled by so much food worked fine; she refused to give in to it. For me, it was difficult; I tried to elicit her support.

"Mom, can we not have so much to eat?"

"No, honey. People expect food at parties."

"I know; but we have enough for a small nation. It's too tempting."

"Don't worry sweetie, it'll get eaten."

"What concerns me is by whom."

Inevitably, there would be "one last thing" that we forgot to put on the table. Surveying the scenery of soups, slaws, and salads, she would exclaim, "We don't have potato salad!"

"Mom, there's plenty. No more, please!"

"Nonsense. Everyone loves potato salad."

"This is a party in my honor, can't we please do it my way?"

"It is for you — but I'm the hostess. We'll do it right."

(The irony is the potato salad was always thrown out later, untouched; a lesson that remained unlearned.)

It annoyed me that she ignored my requests, making it more demanding for me to watch my weight at what was MY party. I know, on the grand scale of things, it's no big deal. But sometimes "little things" get under your skin. It seemed in-considerate. I resented it.

Ruth Marcus would have turned 81 this week. If she were still alive, I would have ecstatically delivered truckloads of potato salad anywhere she wanted me to.

Some things are simply more significant than a perfect diet.

The perfect gift

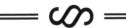

I have trouble accepting that a "lightweight, high power vacuum cleaner" is re-ally the "perfect gift" for Mom, even if — "But wait, there's more!" — they throw in the "super-compact, handy-dandy spot cleaner" when ordered in the next ten minutes.

"Merry Christmas, Mom. How about cleaning the carpets?"

It doesn't ring "holiday spirit" to me; maybe I'm a Grinch.

I am dubious that a pair of shiny, brushed aluminum, "decision dice" — with no shipping charges if ordered today — is the ultimate present for indecisive family members. With a flick of the wrist, they suggest "never" or "think hard." Yet, it doesn't seem the best idea to show Aunt Martha I was thinking of her during Hanukkah.

Although I dispute the claim that the "Cat Lady Action Figure" is the ideal present for the pet lover on my list, I find it humorous, possibly because my wife is a "cat lover" and that toy would provide me with fodder for playful teasing. Unfortunately, "ideal presents" do not include repercussions causing me to have to sleep on the couch, so I scratch it off my list.

"Perfect" is unattainable. Therefore, I now present a few gifts that LEAST serve dieters' needs:

- Tins of cookies, nuts, or fudge. I would not give wine to Uncle Al, celebrating his three years of sobriety; why provide similar temptation to one learning to control his eating? I say I'll only "have a taste," but it's an amazing coincidence that the size of that taste exactly matches the amount in the container. Add to that a hangover of guilt and shame and this is not a good present for me.

- Loose fitting clothes. After a month of excess consumption, what I need most is to regain control, not soft, cushy, expandable-waist sweatpants. In less-controlled days, I was even inclined to don a cheerfully decorated, flowery Hawaiian Mumu come December's end. If it didn't clash so terribly with my tie, I might have taken the leap. A belt is a better idea.

- Another remote control. It's tough enough to fight the coach potato syndrome when it's warm, let alone when the sky is dreary and the sidewalk is soaked. Place a remote in my hand and a brightly flickering 42-inch plasma screen in front of my face, and the recliner will simply swallow me whole. My first step in my new year's exercise plan could be shutting off the TV.

Reality is that the perfect gift is not purchased via cash or credit card, nor wrapped in shiny red boxes topping with sparkling bows. The perfect gift would be the tranquility of self-confidence, the blessing excellent health, the joy of a happy family, and peace and abundance for each person on Earth.

I assure you no one would return that. Happy Holidays.

DEAR SANTA,

You might think I'm a little old to be crawling up on your lap; and after a bulging feast of turkey, mashed potatoes, and uncountable red and green cookies, you probably don't want me weighing down your knee for too long. However, my inner child never grew up; he simply became wrinkled; so I still like some gift requests I have not had answered. I figure, who better than you to help?

I promise I won't take too much time; I understand you're busy and have a few things on your mind. If you prefer, I can email or text my list to your phone; I'm all about the convenience.

First up: I want zero-calorie, great tasting, perfectly textured comfort foods. It is way wrong that when I'm upset, everything I desire causes a weight gain. I get stressed so I eat something comforting. I get fatter — and that stresses me out even more. What's that about? How fair is that? If you can't deliver non-fattening comfort foods, I'll consider the option of modified lettuce that tastes like chocolate. Just a thought…

When I look in the mirror, I want a flat profile looking back; one that doesn't require me sucking in my stomach so deep my voice jumps two octaves. I know, I know; fifty-somethings don't look like 18-year-olds; don't bore me with logic. But in all fairness, I never had the flat, rock hard look as a teenager either, so I'd appreciate seeing what it feels like to have six-pack abs without having to forego the six packs — if you catch my drift. Please don't misunderstand; don't give me a gym membership or sit-up machine; those involve exertion, and who in their right mind wants to wake up Christmas morning to a present requiring sweating and groaning? Yick! I just want to go to sleep chubby, and wake up slim. You figure out how please.

Finally, I want an unending supply of willpower. You can wrap it up in names like "self control" or "determination" if that makes it easier but I'm looking for the ability to resist temptation anytime and whenever it rears its obnoxious green head. Each occasion, I shall make the absolute perfect decision without the raucous, riotous, rambunctious, mental melee that takes place between my ears a thousand times a day. I have important work to do; weighing out the options of whether or not to eat the do-nuts in the work break room is just too darn distracting. Surely, there's something in your woolly red bag to give me the strength to do the right thing every time.

As you can see, there are neither ponies nor sold-out video game consoles in my list, so I'm hoping filling my desires will be trouble-free. And as a thank you, help yourself to some of those chocolate lettuce-flavored zero-calorie cookies. They might not taste as good as the real thing; but — let's be honest — you need to be taking care of your health too.

EMBRACING
THE HERE AND MEOW

Somebody said, "Dogs have masters, cats have staff."

Being a staff member for two cats, I will testify to the veracity of the statement. Our 12-year-old cat, K.C. (um, short for "kitty cat"), has abruptly made a significant behavioral switch, leaving me in the position of having to adjust to this alteration — as I seem powerless in my attempts to convince her to revert to old behaviors. It appears that the bedroom where she has spent many years sleeping, purring — and shedding — is no longer acceptable to wile away the hours. Rather, she has commandeered our bathroom.

In addition to the fact that she has no need for such facilities, I find it puzzling, as tile and porcelain seem to be rather uncomfortable furnishings (especially compared with the warmth and comfort of a carpeted bedroom).

Yet, undeterred by my urgings to return to a softer habitat, she has taken over, napping in the tub or sleeping on the toilet lid. At first I was unnerved in the wee, dark, quiet hours of the night should I happen to sleepishly stagger into the bathroom and be greeted unexpectedly by a low, rumbling, noisy purr. Now, I have learned to simply lift her from the toilet seat, place her on the edge of the tub, take care of business, return her to the lid, pat her good night, and totter unsteadily back to bed. Shaving has become virtually impossible as she jumps onto the vanity and sticks her face in mine. We have developed a dance: I place her on the floor, shave as quickly as possible before she leaps back, re-place her on floor, shave, floor, shave, repeat as necessary.

As with most change, I do eventually adjust.

This is just one aspect of life beyond my control. Should they all be as benign as modifying my morning constitutional to accommodate a furry, affectionate feline, life would be delightful. Yet, that is not so. Often, change crashes in, an out-of-control 18-wheeler through a tent, crushing and crunching everything in its wake; proof of the observation, "Life is what happens while we make other plans."

The question is not, "Will life change?" Instead, it is "How will I adjust to its changes?" Rather than dig in my heels to be dragged screamingly into the dark places, I can find some peace in accepting that the only constant is change. Lamenting a changing diet or the aging of my body does nothing more than tear down my attitude, depleting what I joy I could have.

Change is in all things: the blooming of spring flowers, the laughter of an infant, even the wrinkles around my eyes. It is neither "bad" nor "good," it merely "is."

Embrace it. Adjust to it. And, oh yes, take some time to purr.

WHY WAIT?

When I was a pup, a coveted "grown up treat" was staying up with my father to watch "Gunsmoke," (the longest running weekly TV show in history; 655 episodes from 1955-1975 for trivia buffs).

The character of Festus Haggen, performed by Ken Curtis, was an unusual fellow, whose entire family may have possessed "fewer than 32 teeth among them," as described by one reviewer. He was Illiterate, habitually incoherent, and fiercely loyal to Marshall Dillon, whom he considered one of his two best friends (the other was his mule). During one particularly grueling episode Festus exclaimed, "I wish it was Sunday so I could take a bath!"

Confused, I questioned my father, "Why can't he take a bath today?"

"He only bathes on Sundays."

"What if he gets dirty on Monday or Thursday?"

Replied my impatient father, "Do you want to watch the show or go to bed?" (Which was his not-so-subtle way of saying, "Be quiet.")

As the world turns (no TV reference implied but I admit I'm pleased with utilizing the phrase), we arrive at yet another January, providing many an opportunity to put into action long delayed changes; saying, in effect, "I'm glad it's the New Year so I can finally lose weight."

I admire anyone beginning the punishing pathway to personal

reconstruction; however, why the preoccupation with repeating a pattern every January first, only to give up like a nervous TV executive canceling a sit-com two weeks into its schedule? Yes, January makes sense; a new year is an excellent time to reaffirm direction for life's coming chapter. Yet, it is merely another earthly revolution around its axis. Choose any of 365.

For example, Korean New Year, Hangul, is the first day of their lunar calendar, and the most important of the traditional Korean holidays, lasting three days. It usually occurs in February, providing a refreshed opportunity for resolve just as motivation and the hectic pace of the American holidays begin to wane. Why not start early February?

Or, what about Gudi Padwa, one of the most auspicious days of the Hindu year, believed to be the day that Lord Brahma created the world? In that culture, it is viewed as a time to wipe the slate clean and make a new start, arriving this year in April. Whether that allows us to delay our personal promises three months beyond January or have yet another opportunity to set them in motion is a function of one's determination.

Should April slip past, Rosh Hashanah the beginning of Jewish New Year, is usually celebrated in September. By setting one's vows in the fall, he or she could have a jump start on next year's January rush. It might also be argued that since those two cultures have a combined 10,475 years on their calendars, compared to our 2008, maybe autumn, rather than winter, is more apropos for change?

Selecting specific dates does not ensure the motivation for change will arrive per schedule. To rightly conquer one's demons, experience the enthusiasm of new beginnings, and put to bed the regret of lost days, there is no time like this moment, right now. Should it pass, another opportunity immediately follows; no need to wait.

LOVING THE FLAWS

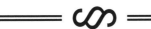

Weight loss is not simply changing one's body; it requires new skills, attitude adjustments, and different means of handling close relationships. Old friends, who have developed patterns over years, now must shift to accommodate new behaviors. Others, unaware of the history, can unintentionally trigger setbacks. Learning to communicate is essential.

When my mother, at age 69, decided to lose the weight she had carried since childhood, she chose an approach that involved changing her food options as minimally as possible; as it was essential to her to maintain a pantry chock full of treats. Therefore any house guest would be served lavishly rich desserts of every fashion. She, however, limited herself to "a taste or two," maintaining a sense of control, but never forsaking dessert. Anyone who had the pleasure of her company understood a meal at Ruth's place was incomplete without dessert; resistance was useless, accept the inevitable. For her, the resultant unhurried pace of weight loss was well worth the sugary gratification following every meal, as surely as the moon must follow the sun.

There is no correct or incorrect dieting style, simply consequences of choices. Choose healthy behaviors; stick with them; accept the results. She did; and lost 80 pounds — over three years.

Upon achieving a healthful weight, yet embarrassed by how much she had previously carried, she wrapped her story of dieting in silence, telling no one who did not know her previously of her astounding success.

At 73, she and Joe began "courting," as he called it. (She explained the relationship as "friends.") Unaware of her weight battles, but having been to her apartment and acutely aware of "The Closet of Sweets," Joe opted to surprise her one afternoon with a dozen fresh, warm donuts, packed neatly in a pink pastry carton. Carrying the gift to her apartment, he rang the doorbell, opened the box, and waited.

The shocker was his. Upon eyeing the pastries, she questioned sharply, "Who are those for?"

"You," he replied, proud of his thoughtfulness.

"Aren't you aware how much I love donuts?" she exclaimed.

"Well, yes, that's why I brought them."

"How could you do this to me?!" she continued, obviously agitated by his actions. "You bring me donuts — knowing how much I like dessert?"

Confused, he stammered, "Uh, yeah, I thought it was a nice thing to do."

"You call that nice – bringing me something I'll eat?!" With that, she slammed hard the door, leaving Joe, perplexed and uncertain in the apartment corridor, kept company by 13 warm donuts.

My mother, normally a very communicative type, held back what she needed for success, feeling humiliated by her past instead of empowered by her achievements.

Releasing shame builds closer relationships and encourages support; our blemishes and imperfections are of small concern to those who love us, glaring large only to ourselves. Acknowledging our flaws actually provides an opportunity to improve and experience a greater level of joy; something especially important this time of year.

Ruth Marcus would have turned 82 this week. Happy Birthday mom; I avoided donuts in your honor.

Made in the USA
Charleston, SC
12 April 2014